Heart Failure: Epidemiology and Research Methods

Heart Failure: Epidemiology and Research Methods

LONGJIAN LIU, MD, PHD, MSC (LSHTM), FAHA
Associate Professor of Eidemiology and Biostatistics
Department of Epidemiology and Biostatistics
Dornsife School of Public Health
Drexel University
Philadelphia, Pennsylvania
and
Adjunct Associate Professor of Medicine,
College of Medicine
Drexel University
Philadelphia, Pennsylvania

ELSEVIER

ELSEVIER

3251 Riverport Lane
St. Louis, Missouri 63043

Content Strategist: Kayla Wolfe
Content Development Manager: Taylor Ball
Publishing Services Manager: Deepthi Unni
Project Manager: Janish Ashwin Paul
Designer: Gopalakrishnan Venkatraman

Printed in United States of America

Last digit is the print number: 9 8 7 6 5 4 3 2 1

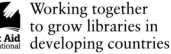

Preface

After my training in preventive medicine, I became interested in clinical epidemiology and biostatistics. My research experience in cardiovascular disease epidemiology and prevention began in 1992, while I was in the MSc program in epidemiology at the London School of Hygiene and Tropical Medicine and had an internship on Cardiovascular Disease and Diabetes Mellitus Epidemiology at the Cambridge University Institute of Public Health. The training and research experience opened up a new and exciting world to me.

In my academic career, from a preventive medicine physician to a tenured professor, I have taught in colleges and schools of medicine and public health for undergraduate and graduate students and have collaborated in local, national, and international research for more than 25 years. This book is a culmination of my teaching and research experience. It is designed for medical students and fellows, public health students, and researchers who are interested in heart failure epidemiology. It also serves as a quick reference guide for students studying cardiovascular disease epidemiology.

This book includes six chapters. Chapter 1 focuses on the basic concepts of cardiology, preventive cardiology, principles of epidemiology, cardiovascular disease epidemiology, heart failure epidemiology, and guidelines for heart failure prevention and treatment and provides an outline of research methods. Chapter 2 discusses the pathophysiology and risk factors of heart failure. Chapter 3 covers standard epidemiologic study designs, from ecologic studies to clinical and community trials. Chapter 3 also presents several important data sources that are publicly available for secondary analysis to develop and test new research hypotheses in heart failure and cardiovascular disease epidemiology. Chapter 4 discusses the basic concepts of descriptive and analytical biostatistics. It includes examples of data analysis and interpretation using sample data and Statistical Analysis System (SAS) software, one of the most popular analytic software packages. Chapter 5 discusses advanced analysis methods, including correlation and regression techniques, logistic regression modeling, and survival analysis (GENMOD, Kaplan Meier, and Cox proportional hazards regression modeling). Each example analysis, starting with a research question, is performed using a hands-on approach. SAS programs are provided in detail for each analysis. Finally, Chapter 6 discusses the areas for further research in heart failure epidemiology and prevention.

Several aspects of this book make it a unique contribution to the field of cardiovascular epidemiology. First, it not only focuses on the concepts and study designs applied in heart failure epidemiology but is also relevant to cardiovascular disease epidemiology and prevention. Second, this book emphasizes applied biostatistics, including data analysis strategies, and covers approaches ranging from descriptive analysis to advanced modeling. Finally, it addresses practice issues and provides hands-on training throughout the book using sample datasets and SAS programs (these samples are available upon request. Please contact me at LL85@Drexel.edu. I will get back to you immediately). This book can be used as a course textbook as well as for self-study.

Readers of this book will gain confidence in working with epidemiologic study designs and conducting univariate and multivariate data analyses. This book is the first to combine reading for didactic learning with hands-on practice for those who wish to learn epidemiology and biostatistics in an integrated approach.

Last, but not least, this book is designed and written by the author, which has the advantage of a consistent presentation and coherent interpretation across chapters and sections. Considering that a textbook that integrates epidemiology and biostatistics and focuses on examples of heart failure research has previously not been available, this book is an important contribution to teaching and learning about heart failure. This book may also play a role in stimulating more research and discussion in the new and exciting field of heart failure epidemiology. Meanwhile, I am sure there is room to improve. I welcome and appreciate any comments, queries, and thoughts from readers.

Longjian Liu, MD, PhD, MSc (LSHTM), FAHA
Philadelphia, Pennsylvania
June 2017

Acknowledgments

To my parents, my wife, and my daughter for their encouragement and patients.

To my supervisors and mentors for their inspiration and help in my career training path and their continued support.

To my colleagues and collaborators whom I have been fortunately working together in teaching and research nationwide and worldwide.

My specific appreciation goes to my students too. Without the opportunities they provided me in teaching, mentoring, and working together, it would be impossible for me to write the book with experience, knowledge, and practice.

Longjian Liu, MD, PhD, MSc (LSHTM), FAHA
Philadelphia, Pennsylvania
June 2017

Contents

CHAPTER 1

Introduction

CARDIOLOGY, PREVENTIVE CARDIOLOGY, AND CARDIOVASCULAR DISEASE EPIDEMIOLOGY

Basic Concepts

Cardiology

Cardiology (from Greek καρδιά *kardiā*, "heart," and -λογία *-logia*, "study") is a branch of medicine. It deals with disorders of the heart as well as parts of the circulatory system. It includes medical diagnosis and treatment of coronary heart disease (CHD), heart failure, congenital heart defects, valvular heart disease, and electrophysiology.[1] Today, in clinical practice of cardiology, it covers several standard and new contents, including, but not limited to, acute coronary syndromes, anticoagulation management, arrhythmias, cardiac surgery, cardiooncology, congenital heart disease and pediatric cardiology, diabetes and cardiometabolic disease, dyslipidemia, geriatric cardiology, heart failure, and cardiomyopathies. In the context of the epidemiology of cardiology, it covers almost all these aspects but focuses on etiologic studies, prevention, quality of life, quality of care, and health promotion at population and community levels. Heart disease, including CHD and heart failure, is the number one killer of the Americans for decades. Furthermore, partly because of the increasing number of aging population, increasing prevalence of obesity and diabetes, and the reduction of mortality from CHD, heart failure has become one of the new epidemics of cardiovascular diseases (CVDs) in the United States and most industrialized countries worldwide.[2-7]

Preventive cardiology

Preventive cardiology addresses clinical practice and preventive medicine of cardiology in persons at individual and population levels. The goal of preventive cardiology is to prevent CVD and to reduce the burden of CVD in populations and improve the quality of life and life expectancy in individuals with CVD. In the clinical context, it mainly focuses on (1) patients with established atherosclerotic disease, (2) patients with a subclinical status of the CVD, and (3) patients at high multifactorial risk of developing CVD. Traditionally, physicians focus on more clinical practice with a particular disease. Today, physicians also play a role in preventive practice to respond of the saying, "Prevention is better than Cure." In addition, many hospitals have established preventive cardiology clinics or cardiovascular prevention programs in the United States and other countries. Most countries have preventive cardiology professional societies, which provide an important forum to have health professionals and policy makers work together for control and prevention of CVD. For example, The American Society of Preventive Cardiology (ASPC) aims "to promote the prevention of cardiovascular disease, advocate for the preservation of cardiovascular health, and disseminate high-quality, evidence-based information through the education of healthcare clinicians and their patients"[8] and the European Society of Preventive Cardiology (ESPC) aims "to reduce the burden of cardiovascular disease."[9]

Epidemiology

Epidemiology, as a medicine discipline, has been in existence for over 150 years. Most agree that modern epidemiology started in the 1850s in the United Kingdom from the control of cholera outbreak in the center of London by Dr. John Snow. He applied a systematic and data-driven approach to examine the pattern of the disease distribution and the possible cause of the epidemic of cholera and provided evidence for the control and prevention of cholera at individual persons and community levels in the central London and across the United Kingdom.[10]

Overall, since the 1850s, the contexts of epidemiology have experienced four major theories that have contributed to the development of epidemiology.

The theory of "miasma"

The theory of "miasma" may initially come from the investigation of cholera in the United Kingdom. As shown, there was an underlying "natural law" linking infection with the risk of cholera inversely to the elevation of the soil among residents who lived in the city of London. The lower the elevation where persons lived in, the higher the incidence and mortality of cholera they had. It was hypothesized that "the concentration of miasma, the airborne organic particles, resulting from these processes, was greatest at a lower elevation," which was likely the cause of the epidemic of cholera in London.[11] Although it was an error or "misleading" theory that claimed the epidemic of cholera was because of "bad air," it let, to some degrees, John Snow to question and detect that the contaminated drinking water might be the cause of the epidemic of cholera in London. Under the influence of "miasma" theory, sanitary statistics was developed and played a role in the development of epidemiologic approaches to data collection, comparison, and interpretation in the 1850s. Most agree that these earlier statistics forms that recorded the incidence and mortality from cholera by age, sex, time, and locations are the prime of the *International Classification of Disease* (*ICD*), which we have used and developed until the current version of *ICD-10*.

Theory of bacteriology

In the early 1880s, Robert Koch discovered the tubercle bacillus (1882) and the cholera bacillus (1883). An important era in the development of epidemiology occurred with a particularly deriving identification of specific agents of disease and inferences of cause-effect association in infectious diseases. Koch's postulates became famous in infectious disease studies. The postulates of proving the cause of disease should include the following. (1) A specific microorganism is present in all cases of the disease. (2) The organism can be obtained in pure culture outside the host (i.e., the individuals with the disease). (3) The organism, when inoculated into a susceptible host (such as an animal model), causes the same disease symptoms. (4) The organism can be isolated in pure culture from the experimentally infected host.

Black box theory

Black box theory occurred around the mid-1900s when the chronic disease has become one of the main burdens of disease. However, the cause of the chronic disease was largely unknown, like a "black box," a system of which the input and output are known but of which nothing is known about what happens inside.[12] For example, using Koch's theory (i.e., postulates), it is unable to detect the cause of chronic disease because no specific bacteria could be detected in patients with chronic disease. There must be new causes rather than bacteria that lead to the development of chronic disease. In the mid-1900s in the United Kingdom, Richard Doll and A. Bradford Hill conducted a population-based prospective study to investigate whether smoking was a risk factor for the development of lung cancer among British doctors. It becomes one of the major milestones of the development of noncommunicable disease epidemiology.

In 1948, the US National Heart Institute (now known as the National Heart, Lung, and Blood Institute) supported the first largest cardiovascular epidemiology study, the Framingham Heart Study. At the early time, like the cause of cancer, little was known about the cause of heart disease and stroke.

System theory

It was around the early 1980s. New knowledge of the understanding of the complex disease at the microlevel (genomic and molecular) and macrolevel (lifestyle, behaviors, environmental and social determinants) are significantly improved. The revolutionary development of new technology and research tools, including the revolutionary development of computer and biostatistics software, makes it possible to investigate the cause of disease using a systematic approach.

Since the 1900s, the patterns of leading cause of deaths have dramatically changed from communicable disease to noncommunicable disease. Epidemiology of noncommunicable disease was developed. It plays a pivotal role in chronic disease control and prevention and becomes a major discipline in epidemiology research and education.[13]

Principles of epidemiology

The principles of epidemiology include study designs, testing research hypotheses, exploring possible causal associations between risk factors (i.e., exposures) and outcomes, and addressing disease control and prevention. It plays a fundamental role in medicine and public health. Epidemiology, by the definition endorsed by the International Association of Epidemiology, is "the study of the occurrence and distribution of health-related events, states, and processes in specified populations, including the study of the determinants influencing such processes, and the application of this knowledge to control relevant health problems."[14] What is noteworthy about this definition is that it includes both a description of the content of the discipline and the purpose or application for which epidemiologic investigations are carried out.[11] The distribution of health-related states or events in specified populations can be outlined by three "W's," Who, When, and Where. In Figs. 1.1–1.3, we used data from the US Centers for Disease Control and Prevention (CDC)—Wide-ranging ONline Data for Epidemiologic Research (CDC WONDER) to demonstrate few examples of the three "W's" applications.[15]

Who are attacked by the disease?. Fig. 1.1 depicts the trend of age-specific mortality rates (per 100,000) from heart failure in people aged 35 and older (Fig. 1.1A) and in those aged 65 and older (Fig. 1.1B) by sex in the United States during the period 2013–2015. It indicates that males had a higher risk of mortality from

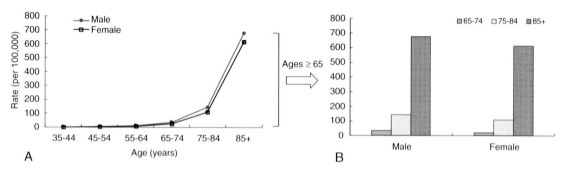

FIG. 1.1 Age-adjusted mortality (per 100,000) from heart failure by sex and age in people aged 35 and older **(A)**, and people aged 65 and older **(B)** in the United States during the period 2013–2015. (Data from CDC WONDER.)

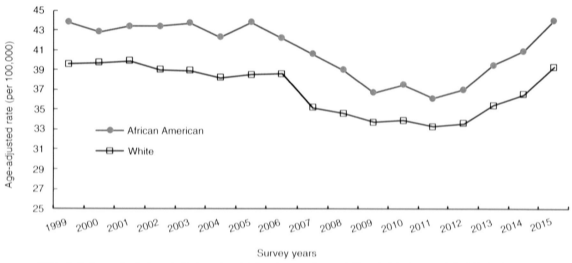

FIG. 1.2 Age-adjusted mortality from heart failure in people aged 35 and older by race/ethnicity in the United States from 1999 to 2015. (Data from CDC WONDER.)

heart failure than females by each age group (Fig. 1.1A), and the mortality increases from those aged 65 and older, with an especially sharp increase in people aged 85 and older in both males and females (Fig. 1.1B).

When did/does the disease change its pattern or when did/does the disease occur? Fig. 1.2 depicts the trend of age-adjusted mortality (per 100,000) from heart failure in white and African Americans aged 35 and older from 1999 to 2015 in the United States. It suggests that African Americans had higher age-adjusted mortality rates from heart failure than whites during the period 1999–2015, and there was a dramatically decreasing trend from 2005 to 2011 and then an increasing trend from 2012 to 2015 in the mortality among both white and African Americans in the United States.

Where did/does the disease exist and/or have?. Fig. 1.3 depicts the trend of age-adjusted mortality rates in patients with heart failure aged 35 and older by states in the United States during the period 2013–2015. It indicates that there were huge variations in mortality rates from heart failure across the states. Of the top five, the state of Mississippi had the highest age-adjusted mortality rates (85 per 100,000 population), followed by Alabama (84.7 per 100,000 population), Louisiana (71.2 per 100,000 population), Utah (68.4 per 100,000 population), and Georgia (59.3 per 100,000 population) in 2013–2015.

Regarding epidemiologic research approaches, it has two overall approves: one is called descriptive epidemiology (i.e., the description of three "W's"), and the other is called analytical epidemiology. In descriptive epidemiology, investigators describe the burden of

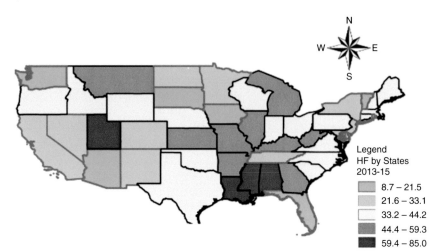

FIG. 1.3 Age-adjusted mortality rates (per 100,000 population) from heart failure in people aged 35 and older by states in the United States during the period 2013–2015. (Data from CDC WONDER.)

disease and/or risk factors and generate research questions for further studies through analytical epidemiology that it aims to examine 'Why? and How?"

Cardiovascular Disease Epidemiology

CVD epidemiology is a branch of chronic epidemiology and public health. It involves the understanding of the causes of CVDs, identification of methods of prevention, and monitoring of populations to assess the changing burden of CVDs and the measurable impact of interventions to control these diseases.[16]

CVD epidemiology addresses a broader group of disorders of the heart and blood vessels compared with clinical cardiology. Studies of CVD epidemiology commonly includes six major forms of diseases related to heart and blood vessels: (1) CHD, (2) stroke, (3) heart failure, (4) peripheral arterial disease, (5) rheumatic heart disease, and (6) congenital heart disease.

In addition, using the codes of the *ICD* for CVDs, hypertension is also one of the major types of CVDs. However, we commonly study hypertension as a single disease only, or as a risk factor for heart disease, stroke, and other high blood pressure–related disease in epidemiologic studies.

Examples of cardiovascular disease epidemiology

Framingham Heart Study. The US Framingham Heart Study (FHS), initiated in 1947, is one of the earliest cardiovascular epidemiologic studies that focus on the causes of CVD, distribution, and prevention of this disease at a population level.[17]

WHO MONICA Study. Since the early 1980s, several national and international studies in CVD epidemiology

and prevention have been conducted. The World Health Organization (WHO) MONICA (Monitoring Trends and Determinants in Cardiovascular Disease) Study was one of the largest international collaborative studies, including 32 collaborating centers in 21 counties. Exposures to cigarette smoking, high blood pressure, serum or plasma total cholesterol and high-density lipoprotein cholesterol, and body mass index (=weight [kg]/height [m^2]) were four key measures in the WHO MONICA study.[18]

The Atherosclerosis Risk in Communities Study. The Atherosclerosis Risk in Communities (ARIC) Study is a prospective study to investigate the etiology of atherosclerosis and its clinical sequelae and variation in cardiovascular risk factors, medical care, and disease by race, sex, place, and time, in each of four US communities—Forsyth County, North Carolina; Jackson, Mississippi; suburbs of Minneapolis, Minnesota; and Washington County, Maryland.[19]

The Cardiovascular Health Study. The Cardiovascular Health Study (CHS) is a population-based, longitudinal study of CHD and stroke in adults aged 65 years and older. The main objective of the study is to identify factors related to the onset and course of CHD and stroke. CHS is designed to determine the importance of conventional CVD risk factors in older adults and to identify new risk factors in this age group, especially those that may be protective and modifiable. The study design called for enrollment of 1250 men and women in each of four communities: Forsyth County, North Carolina; Sacramento County, California; Washington County, Maryland; and Pittsburgh, Pennsylvania. Eligible participants were sampled from Medicare eligibility lists in each area.[20]

The WHO-CARDIAC Study. The WHO-coordinated Cardiovascular Disease Alimentary Comparison Study (WHO-CARDIAC Study) was designed to examine the associations of biomarkers from urine and blood samples with blood pressure, and risk of mortality from CHD and stroke. It included more than 60 collaborative centers from 25 countries worldwide.[21-23]

The Jackson Heart Study. The purposes of the Jackson Heart Study are to (1) establish a single-site cohort study to identify the risk factors for the development of CVDs, especially those related to hypertension, in African American men and women; (2) build research capabilities in minority institutions by building partnerships; (3) attract minority students to careers in public health and epidemiology; and (4) establish an NHLBI (National Heart, Lung, and Blood Institute) Field Site in Jackson, Mississippi, similar to those established for the Framingham Heart Study and the Honolulu Heart Program.[24]

The Multi-Ethnic Study of Atherosclerosis. The Multi-Ethnic Study of Atherosclerosis (MESA) is a prospective cohort study of men and women aged 45–84 years without a history of the clinical CVD living in six US communities. These communities include Baltimore; Chicago; Forsyth County, North Carolina; Los Angeles County, California; New York City; and St. Paul, Minnesota. The study objective of MESA is to identify risk factors for subclinical CVD, for progression of subclinical CVD, and for transition from subclinical to clinical CVD.[25-27]

Significance

CVDs are the leading cause of morbidity and mortality in the United States. In 2010, CVD was a primary diagnosis for more than 7.8 million inpatients hospital discharges and 4.6 million emergency department encounters. Although CVD death rates have declined over the past decades, it remains the leading cause of death. It accounted for 30.6% of all death, with heart disease still the first, and strokes the fourth leading causes of death in the United States in 2014.[28,29]

EPIDEMIOLOGY OF HEART FAILURE: NEW INSIGHTS INTO RESEARCH AND PREVENTION

Basic Concepts

Heart failure, one of the major forms of CVDs, is a complex clinical syndrome. It can result from any structural or functional cardiac disorder that impairs the ability of the ventricle to fill with or eject blood. The cardinal manifestations of HF are dyspnea and fatigue, which may limit exercise tolerance, and fluid retention, which may lead to pulmonary and/or splanchnic congestion and/or peripheral edema. It should be noted that some patients may have exercise intolerance but little evidence of fluid retention, whereas others complain primarily of edema, dyspnea, or fatigue, or some patients present without signs or symptoms of volume overload.[30]

Heart failure is a global pandemic affecting an estimated 26 million people worldwide and resulting in more than 1 million hospitalizations annually in both the United States and Europe.[31]

The unique aspects of the epidemiology of heart failure in research and healthcare practice include, but not limited to, the following:

- The burden of the disease has increased dramatically, with severe impacts on the elderly and underserved populations.
- The differences and changes in the spectrums of the pathways of high blood pressure, hypertrophy, and ventricular systolic and diastolic dysfunctions and outcomes vary by ages, sex, race/ethnicities, and regions.
- The complex disease with comorbidities of hypertension, arrhythmia, coronary arterial disease, renal dysfunction, diabetes mellitus, and lung disease.
- The significantly high readmission rates with complex causes of both pathophysiologic and socioeconomic determinants.
- The complex disease with multiple medications and drug-drug, and drug-environmental interactions.

Epidemiology of Heart Failure

Heart failure poses a serious health issues in old adults

In the United States, about 5.7 million adults have heart failure, and there are 670,000 new cases in every single year. About half of people who develop heart failure die within 5 years of diagnosis. Heart failure costs the nation an estimated $30.7 billion each year. This total includes the cost of healthcare services, medications to treat heart failure, and missed days of work.[32,33]

Heart failure disproportionally affects the elderly, starting in those aged 65 and older. Most patients with heart failure are more than 75 years of age, and approximately half of these will die within a year of hospital admission. Of patients aged less than 75 years, about one in five will die within a year of admission.[4,34]

Fig. 1.1 depicts that heart failure mortality rates increase dramatically in people aged 65 and older, with a specifically increasing in those aged 75 and older (Fig. 1.1). It is the leading killer of the elderly.

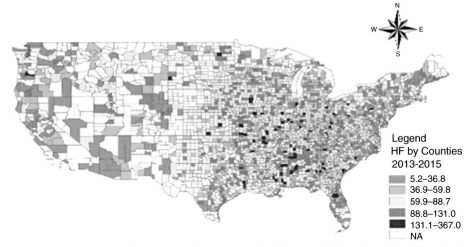

FIG. 1.4 Age-adjusted mortality rates (per 100,000 population) from heart failure in people aged 35 and older by counties in the United States during the period 2013–2015. (Data from CDC WONDER. NA: Data not available)

Heart failure mortality rates increase in recent years

Although there was a decreased trend in age-adjusted heart failure mortality from 1999 to 2009, the rates increase again from around 2011 to 2015 in both white and African Americans in the United States. Age-adjusted mortality from heart failure were continuously higher in African Americans than whites (Fig. 1.2).

Heart failure mortality rates vary by states in the United States

Heart failure mortality rates vary by states, with higher rates in southeastern states (Fig. 1.3).

Similar to the state level, there are significant variations in heart failure mortality across counties in the United States (Fig. 1.4).

Trends of heart failure

Since the early 1980s, heart failure has been emerging as a significant public health concern because of its increasing trends in incidence, prevalence, and mortality.

Fig. 1.5 shows that of the three major forms of CVD (heart failure, coronary heart disease, and cerebra-vascular disease), age-adjusted prevalence of hospitalization from heart failure in patients aged 65 and older who had a primary diagnosis of the disease increased in whites (Fig. 1.5 left side) and in African Americans (right side), with a specific increasing trend in African Americans from 1995 to 2010 in the United States.

Heart failure represents a new epidemic of CVD, affecting about 5.7 million Americans aged 20 and older (NHANES 2009–12). It is estimated that about 915,000 new heart failure cases occur annually according to data from ARIC 2002–2012.[28] In 2013, any-mention mortality was 300,122 (140,126 males and 159,996 females), and heart failure was the underlying cause in 65,120 of those deaths.[28] In contrast to other CVDs, the prevalence, incidence, and mortality from heart failure are increasing, and prognosis remains poor.[4,5,35]

Increased mortality rate in young adults

Fig. 1.6 depicts an increasing trend in age-specific mortality rates in US young adults aged 35–64 from 2001–03 to 2013–15 (A) and a decreased trend in the older adults (B).

Increased trend in multiple comorbidities

Multiple comorbidities in patients with heart have raised an even complication issue in both etiologic study and healthcare practice. Fig. 1.7 shows that the prevalence of heart failure patients with comorbidities of CHD, chronic obstructive pulmonary disease, and renal failure have increased in recent decades in both sexes, except a slight decrease in comorbidity of cerebrovascular disease.

HFSA AND AHA GUIDELINES FOR HEART FAILURE PREVENTION AND TREATMENT
Basic Concepts

In 1999, the first heart failure guideline was developed by the Heart Failure Society of America (HFSA). It had a narrow scope, concentrating on the pharmacologic

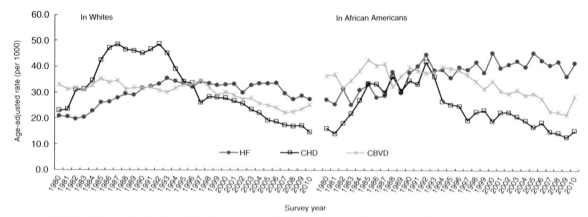

FIG. 1.5 Age-adjusted hospitalization rate (per 1000) in patients with a primary diagnosis of coronary heart disease, or cerebrovascular disease (CBVD), or heart failure by sex from 1980 to 2006 in the United States. (Data from NHDS.)

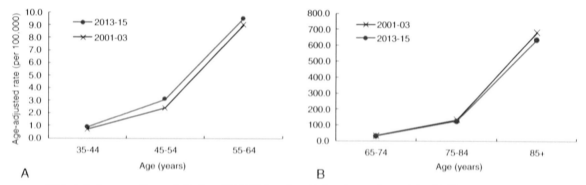

FIG. 1.6 Age-specific mortality (per 100,000) from heart failure in people aged 35–64 **(A)** and those aged 65 and older **(B)** in the United States during five periods of 2001–03 and 2013–15. (Data from WONDER.)

treatment of chronic, symptomatic left ventricular dysfunction.[16,17] The guideline did not consider subsets of the clinical syndrome of heart failure, including acute decompensated heart failure and "diastolic dysfunction," or prevention issues.[17] In 2006 and 2009, two following comprehensive clinical practice guidelines were published to address a full range of topics, including prevention, evaluation, disease management, and pharmacologic and device therapy for patients with heart failure, and add a section on the genetic evaluation of cardiomyopathy.[18,19] In 2010, HFSA updated and expanded each of these areas.[17] Furthermore, since 2001 the American College of Cardiology Foundation (ACCF) and the American Heart Association (AHA) has proposed new classifications of heart failure by A, B, C, and D stages. In the new proposals, prevention and control of heart failure have been paid a considerable attention by clinical cardiologists and most relevant

fields of professional healthcare practitioners.[13,30,40] For example, in 2013, the ACCF and AHA have jointly produced guidelines for the management of heart failure, in which the complexity of the disease with multiple comorbidities, including CHD, chronic kidney disease, and diabetes, have been addressed.[30]

Significance

Today, the knowledge about heart failure clinical epidemiology is accumulating rapidly. Individual physicians may be unable to readily and adequately synthesize new information into effective strategies for care and prevention in patients with heart failure. Data from clinical trials, although they are valuable, often do not give direction for individual patient management and lacks information for patients with heart failure in the general population, which are driven only by population based studies. These characteristics make heart

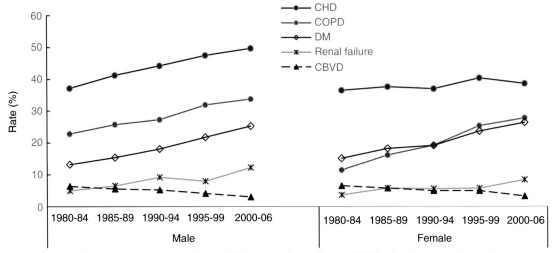

FIG. 1.7 Changes in prevalence of comorbid coronary heart disease (CHD), chronic obstructive pulmonary disease (COPD), diabetes mellitus (DM), renal failure, or cerebrovascular disease (CBVD) in patients with primary diagnosis of heart failure aged 65 and older in males and females from 1980 to 2006 in the United States. (Data from NHDS.)

failure an ideal candidate for practice guidelines in both clinical and community settings. The 2010 HFSA comprehensive practice guideline addresses the full range of evaluation, care, and management of patients with heart failure. This updated HFSA 2010 guideline highlights the importance of control heart failure at primordial, primary, secondary, and tertiary preventions because patients at risk for many CVDs are at risk for heart failure. Early identification and control of risk factors is perhaps the most significant step in limiting the adverse public health impact of heart failure. Emphasis on primordial, primary, and secondary prevention is particularly critical because of the difficulty of treating left ventricular dysfunction successfully, especially when severe. Current therapeutic advances in the treatment of heart failure do not make prevention any less important.[37]

RESEARCH METHODS APPLIED IN HEART FAILURE EPIDEMIOLOGY

Basic Concepts

Research methods refer to descriptive and analytical epidemiologic studies, which include applied biostatistics.

Descriptive epidemiology

Descriptive epidemiology aims to describe the distributions of diseases and determinants. It provides a way of organizing and analyzing these data to describe the variations in disease frequency among populations by geographical areas and over time (i.e., person, place, and time). Descriptive epidemiology can thus generate hypotheses of etiologic research.

Ecologic study and cross-sectional study (see Chapter 4) are the most commonly applied in descriptive epidemiologic studies. For example, the National Health and Nutrition Examination Survey is a cross-sectional study. In the study, participants' health conditions, including the prevalence of CHD, heart failure, stroke, diabetes, and cancers, are measured through standard survey instruments.[41]

Analytical epidemiology

Analytical epidemiology aims to study the associations between exposures (i.e., risk and protective factors of diseases) and outcomes (i.e., incidence, prevalence, and mortality). Analytical epidemiology can thus test research hypotheses of potentially causality effects and/or associations between exposures and outcomes.

Analytical epidemiology study design includes observational studies (case-control and cohort studies) and experimental studies (clinical and community trials). Data analysis for a study with analytical epidemiology design includes the following:

- Test rate and proportion differences using chi-square test, logistic regression, and Cox proportional hazard regression models (see Chapter 4)
- Test mean differences using student t-test, analysis of variance (ANOVA), a simple and partial correlation

between exposures and outcomes, and simple and multiple regression models (see Chapter 4)

New Research and Analysis Approaches Applied in Heart Failure Study

With the advances in standard computer software and biostatistics methods, several new biostatistics methods are applied in epidemiologic analyses. For example, life course epidemiologic study design and analysis approach have been applied in cardiovascular epidemiologic studies.[42,43] Calculation of propensity score is used to control multiple confounders.[44] Mediation analysis,[45] as well as multilevel regression analysis, is applied to test diffident associations between exposures and outcomes by individuals and small area levels.[46–48] Reduced rank regression (RRR) models are applied to test associations between hypothesis-driven exposures and outcomes.[26,48,49] Quantile regression (QR) techniques are used to address health disparities in studies of cardiovascular risk factors.[50]

Life course epidemiology

Life course epidemiology examines the long-term biological, behavioral, and psychosocial processes that may link risk exposures from early life to adult life across the whole life span. In the early life, it can be back to Barker's fetal origins hypothesis in the mid-1980s.[51] David Barber's studies on maternal nutrition, birth weight, and risk of CVD mortality in late life are the earlier examples using life course epidemiologic approach.[43,52] In the 1990s, working with colleagues in the International Agency for Research on Cancer, we identified that women who had poor early-life experience had a higher risk of breast cancer than their corresponding counterparts.[53] In an early study using data from Japan cancer registry, we observed a significantly ecologic association between infant mortality and stroke mortality across counties in Japan.[54] Recently, we analyzed longitudinal data from the US Health and Retirement Study (HRS) to demonstrate that the risk of stroke mortality in adults is significantly associated with subjects who had poor life experience in their early life.[42]

Propensity score

The propensity score is the probability of treatment assignment conditional on observed baseline characteristics. This score allows one to design and analyze an observational (i.e., nonrandomized) study so that it mimics some of the particular characteristics of a randomized controlled trial.[55]

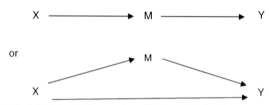

FIG. 1.8 A typical case of mediation analysis. M is a mediator that explains the underlying mechanism of the relationship between X and Y.

Mediation analysis

Mediation is a hypothesized causal chain in which one variable affects the second variable that, in turn, it has an impact on a third variable (Y). Mediation analysis is typically applied when a researcher wants to assess the extent to which the effect of exposure (X) is explained, or is not explained, by a given set of hypothesized mediators (M, also called intermediate variables) (Fig. 1.8).[56,57]

For example, a study found a total effect of metabolic syndrome (yes versus no) on the risk of heart failure equal to a relative risk of 2.5. After adjustment for inflammation factors (such as serum C-reactive protein), the relative risk decreased to 2.0, and the percent excess risk of metabolic syndrome on the risk of heart failure explained by the inflammation status (high versus low) would be 33.3% [(2.5−2.0)/(2.5−1)*100].

It should be noted that we test whether an exposure (X) affects a mediator (M). If there is no relationship between the exposure and mediator (as indicates in Fig. 1.6), the mediator should be treated as a third variable that may or may not be associated with the outcome of interest. It is meaningful to test a mediator only if an exposure affects the mediator of interest.[57]

Multilevel analysis

It is a relatively new statistical technique in epidemiologic research. It can be viewed as a modern way of addressing research questions concerning how outcomes change by individual and small area levels. It is also known as hierarchical linear regression models, nested data models, and mixed models. It addresses that statistical models of parameters of interest vary at more than one level. An example could be an analysis of patients with heart failure whom we measured several biomarkers for individual patients, as well as measures for hospitals within which the patients are grouped. The purpose of the multilevel analysis is to take variations in both individuals and hospitals. This analysis has become popular because more computer

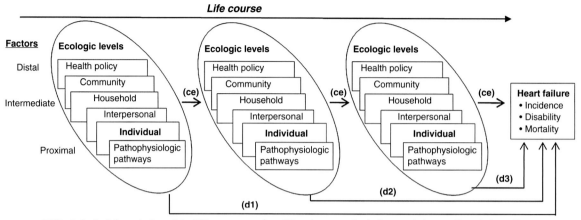

FIG. 1.9 An integrated model of life course and multilevel approach. *(ce)*, cumulative and/or chains effect on outcomes; *(d)*, direct effect across lifespan at different ages; *(d1)*, childhood; *(d2)*, adolescence; *(d3)*, adult life.

software can perform the analysis easily.[46,58] Fig. 1.9 depicts an integrated conceptual model of life course and multilevel approach for the study of risk of heart failure.

Reduced rank regression (RRR) models

RRR model identifies linear functions of predictors that explain as much variation as possible in response variables, which were considered as intermediate markers of the predictors of interest for the study outcomes.[59] RRR model is an innovative technique to establish dietary patterns related to biochemical risk factors for type 2 diabetes and metabolic syndrome. For example, built on a priori knowledge of a biological relationship between a dietary pattern with high process intake and risk of left ventricular dysfunction, to examine whether this relationship is mediated by metabolic syndrome, we identified a dietary pattern that explains as much variation as possible in metabolic syndrome. Results from RRR analysis provides new evidence that the relationship between diet and risk of left ventricular dysfunction is mediated by metabolic disorder.[26]

Quantile regression (QR) techniques

The QR approach assesses how conditional quantiles of the response variable vary with measured covariates. One advantage of the QR, relative to the ordinary least squares regression, is that the QR estimates are more robust against outliers in the response measurements. it provides a complete picture of the conditional distribution than a single estimate of the center estimate that is done using linear regression models.[60] For example, to examine health disparities in CVD risk scores in individuals with chronic kidney disease for African Americans versus whites, we used data from the Chronic Renal Insufficiency Cohort (CRIC) Study and used QR technique in the final data analysis. The results indicate that African Americans had significantly higher CVD risk scores in quantile 4 than whites. This race/ethnicity difference in CVD risk score was even worse among young African Americans (aged <65) than their white counterparts.[61]

Mapping and visualization

Mapping and visualization techniques using data from large scale have been recently applied. Now, several standard software can describe the distributions of disease and determinants using mapping, visualization, and univariate and multivariate analysis techniques, such as SAS, Geographic Information System, SPSS, R, and Stata.

Significance

Standard and new epidemiologic methods have met the challenges facing in heart failure epidemiologic studies. Specifically, standard computer software can conduct general and complex biostatistics efficiently and effectively, and results of biostatistics are easily interpreted and understood. In this textbook, several standard and new data analysis methods are presented step by step and discussed in Chapter 4.

REFERENCES

1. *Wikipedia. Cardiology.* 2016. https://en.wikipedia.org/wiki/Cardiology.
2. Massie BM, Shah NB. The heart failure epidemic: magnitude of the problem and potential mitigating approaches. *Curr Opin Cardiol.* 1996;11(3):221–226.
3. Johansen H, Strauss B, Arnold JMO, Moe G, Liu P. On the rise: The current and projected future burden of congestive heart failure hospitalization in Canada. *Can J Cardiol.* 2003;19(4):430–435.
4. Liu L. Changes in cardiovascular hospitalization and co-morbidity of heart failure in the United States: findings from the National Hospital Discharge Surveys 1980–2006. *Int J Cardiol.* 2011;149(1):39–45.
5. Liu L, Eisen HJ. Epidemiology of heart failure and scope of the problem. *Cardiol Clin.* 2014;32(1):1–8.
6. Masoudi FA, Havranek EP, Krumholz HM. The burden of chronic congestive heart failure in older persons: magnitude and implications for policy and research. *Heart Fail Rev.* 2002;7(1):9–16.
7. Tsao L, Gibson CM. Heart failure: an epidemic of the 21st century. *Crit Pathw Cardiol.* 2004;3(4):194–204.
8. The American Society for Preventive Cardiology. Mission Statement. https://www.aspconline.org/mission-statement.
9. ESPC. European Society of Preventive Cardiology. https://www.escardio.org/The-ESC/Who-we-are.
10. Cameron D, Jones IG. John Snow, the Broad Street pump and modern epidemiology. *Int J Epidemiol.* 1983;12(4):393–396.
11. Gordis L. *Epidemiology.* 5th ed. Toronto, Canada: Elsevier Canada; 2014.
12. Youngson RM. *Collins Dictionary of Medicine Fourth Edition;* 2005.
13. Liu L, Newschaffer CJ, Nelson J. Cardiovascular Disease. In: Remington PL, Brownson RC, Wegner MV, eds. *Chronic Disease Epidemiology and Control.* vol. 4. Washington: American Public Health Association; 2016:673–742.
14. Association IE. *A Dictionary of Epidemiology.* 4th ed. 198 Madison Avenue, New York, NY 10016: Oxford University Press; 2014.
15. CDC WONDER. Wide-ranging online data for epidemiologic research. 1999–2015 Data; https://wonder.cdc.gov/.
16. Labarthe DR. *Epidemiology and Prevention of Cardiovascular Diseases – A Global Challenge.* 2nd ed. Jones and Bartlett Publishers; 2011.
17. Kannel WB, McGee DL. Diabetes and cardiovascular disease. The Framingham study. *JAMA.* 1979;241(19):2035–2038.
18. Kuulasmaa K, Tunstall-Pedoe H, Dobson A, et al. Estimation of contribution of changes in classic risk factors to trends in coronary event rates across the WHO MONICA Project populations. *Lancet.* 2000;355(9205):675–687.
19. Investigators A. The Atherosclerosis Risk in Communities (ARIC) study: design and objectives. *Am J Epidemiol.* 1989;129(4):687–702.
20. Fried LP, Borhani NO, Enright P, et al. The cardiovascular health study: design and rationale. *Ann Epidemiol.* 1991;1(3):263–276.
21. Yamori Y, Liu L, Ikeda K, et al. Distribution of twenty-four hour urinary taurine excretion and association with ischemic heart disease mortality in 24 populations of 16 countries: results from the WHO-CARDIAC Study. *Hypertens Res.* 2001;24(4):453–457.
22. Liu L, Ikeda K, Yamori Y, Group W-CS. Inverse relationship between urinary markers of animal protein intake and blood pressure in Chinese: results from the WHO Cardiovascular Diseases and Alimentary Comparison (CARDIAC) Study. *Int J Epidemiol.* 2002;31(1):227–233.
23. Liu L, Liu L, Ding Y, et al. Ethnic and environmental differences in various markers of dietary intake and blood pressure among Chinese Han and three other minority peoples of China: results from the WHO Cardiovascular Diseases and Alimentary Comparison (CARDIAC) Study. *Hypertens Res.* 2001;24(3):315–322.
24. Sempos CT, Bild DE, Manolio TA. Overview of the Jackson Heart Study: a study of cardiovascular diseases in African American men and women. *Am J Med Sci.* 1999;317(3):142–146.
25. Wong TY, Islam FA, Klein R, et al. Retinal vascular caliber, cardiovascular risk factors, and inflammation: the multi-ethnic study of atherosclerosis (MESA). *Invest Ophthalmol Vis Sci.* 2006;47(6):2341–2350.
26. Liu L, Nettleton JA, Bertoni AG, Bluemke DA, Lima JA, Szklo M. Dietary pattern, the metabolic syndrome, and left ventricular mass and systolic function: the multi-ethnic study of atherosclerosis. *Am J Clin Nutr.* 2009;90(2):362–368.
27. Bild DE, Bluemke DA, Burke GL, et al. Multi-ethnic study of atherosclerosis: objectives and design. *Am J Epidemiol.* 2002;156(9):871–881.
28. Mozaffarian D, Benjamin EJ, Go AS, et al. Heart disease and stroke statistics—2016 update a report from the American Heart Association. *Circulation.* 2015. http://dx.doi.org/10.1161/CIR.0000000000000350.
29. Lloyd-Jones D, Adams R, Carnethon M, et al. Heart disease and stroke statistics—2009 update: a report from the American Heart Association Statistics Committee and Stroke Statistics Subcommittee. *Circulation.* 2009;119(3):480–486.
30. Yancy CW, Jessup M, Bozkurt B, et al. 2013 ACCF/AHA guideline for the management of heart failure. *Circulation.* 2013. http://dx.doi.org/10.1161/CIR.0b013e31829e8776.
31. Ambrosy AP, Fonarow GC, Butler J, et al. The global health and economic burden of hospitalizations for heart failure: lessons learned from hospitalized heart failure registries. *J Am Coll Cardiol.* 2014;63(12):1123–1133.
32. Roger VL, Go AS, Lloyd-Jones DM, et al. Executive summary: heart disease and stroke statistics—2012 update: a report from the American Heart Association. *Circulation.* 2012;125(1):188–197.
33. Heidenreich PA, Albert NM, Allen LA, et al. Forecasting the impact of heart failure in the United States: a policy statement from the American Heart Association. *Circ Heart Fail.* 2013;6(3):606–619.
34. Kosiborod M, Lichtman JH, Heidenreich PA, et al. National trends in outcomes among elderly patients with heart failure. *Am J Med.* 2006;119(7):e616.e611–e616.e617.

35. Hunt SA, Abraham WT, Chin MH, et al. 2009 focused update incorporated into the ACC/AHA 2005 Guidelines for the Diagnosis and Management of Heart Failure in Adults: a report of the American College of Cardiology Foundation/American Heart Association Task Force on Practice Guidelines: developed in collaboration with the International Society for Heart and Lung Transplantation. *Circulation*. 2009;119(14):e391–e479.

36. KF JA, Baughman K, Dec W, et al. HFSA guidelines for the management of patients with heart failure due to left ventricular systolic dysfunction-pharmacological approaches. *Congest Heart Fail*. 2000;6(1).

37. Heart Failure Society of America. Executive summary: HFSA 2010 comprehensive heart failure practice guideline. *J Card Fail*. 2010;16(6):475–539.

38. Heart Failure Society of America. Executive summary: HFSA 2006 comprehensive heart failure practice guideline. *J Card Fail*. 2006;12(1):10–38.

39. Hershberger RE, Lindenfeld J, Mestroni L, Seidman CE, Taylor MR, Towbin JA. Genetic evaluation of cardiomyopathy—a Heart Failure Society of America practice guideline. *J Card Fail*. 2009;15(2):83–97.

40. Hunt SA, Baker DW, Chin MH, et al. ACC/AHA guidelines for the evaluation and management of chronic heart failure in the adult: executive summary: A report of the American College of Cardiology/American Heart Association task force on practice guidelines (committee to revise the 1995 guidelines for the evaluation and management of heart failure) developed in collaboration with the international society for heart and lung transplantation endorsed by the heart failure society of america. *J Am Coll Cardiol*. 2001;38(7):2101–2113.

41. CDC NCHS: National Health and Nutrition Examination Survey, https://www.cdc.gov/nchs/nhanes/index.htm.

42. Liu L, Xue F, Ma J, Ma M, Long Y, Newschaffer CJ. Social position and chronic conditions across the life span and risk of stroke: a life course epidemiological analysis of 22 847 American adults in ages over 50. *Int J Stroke*. 2013;8(A100):50–55.

43. Barker DJ. Fetal nutrition and cardiovascular disease in later life. *Br Med Bull*. 1997;53(1):96–108.

44. Giamouzis G, Sui X, Love TE, Butler J, Young JB, Ahmed A. A propensity-matched study of the association of cardiothoracic ratio with morbidity and mortality in chronic heart failure. *Am J Cardiol*. 2008;101(3):343–347.

45. Stout RL. Advancing the analysis of treatment process. *Addiction (Abingdon, England)*. 2007;102(10):1539–1545.

46. Liu L, Núñez AE. Multilevel and urban health modeling of risk factors for diabetes mellitus: a new insight into public health and preventive medicine. *Adv Prev Med*. 2014;2014.

47. Clark CR, Coull B, Berkman LF, Buring JE, Ridker PM. Geographic variation in cardiovascular inflammation among healthy women in the Women's Health Study. *PLoS One*. 2011;6(11):e27468.

48. Hoffmann K, Schulze MB, Schienkiewitz A, Nothlings U, Boeing H. Application of a new statistical method to derive dietary patterns in nutritional epidemiology. *Am J Epidemiol*. 2004;159(10):935–944.

49. Nettleton JA, Steffen LM, Schulze MB, et al. Associations between markers of subclinical atherosclerosis and dietary patterns derived by principal components analysis and reduced rank regression in the multi-ethnic study of atherosclerosis (MESA). *Am J Clin Nutr*. 2007;85(6):1615–1625.

50. Liu L. *Using Multivariate Quantile Regression Analysis to Explore Cardiovascular Risk Differences in Subjects with Chronic Kidney Disease by Race and Ethnicity: Findings from the US Chronic Renal Insufficiency Cohort Study* Paper presented at: International Cardiovascular Forum Journal. 2015.

51. Ben-Shlomo DKaY. *A Life Course Approach to Chronic Disease Epidemiology*. Great Clarendo Street, Oxford OX2 6DP, UK: Oxford University Press; 2004.

52. Barker DJ, Lackland DT. Prenatal influences on stroke mortality in England and Wales. *Stroke*. 2003;34(7):1598–1602.

53. Liu L, Wu K, Lin X, et al. Passive smoking and other factors at different periods of life and breast cancer risk in Chinese women who have never smoked—a case-control study in Chongqing. People's Republic of China *Asian Pac J Cancer Prev*. 2000;1(2):131–137.

54. Liu Z, Liu L. Infant mortality, cancer, and cardiovascular disease mortality: an ecological analysis for 47 prefectures of Japan. *Int J Cardiol*. 2011;149(2):242–243.

55. Austin PC. An introduction to propensity score methods for reducing the effects of confounding in observational studies. *Multivariate Behav Res*. 2011;46(3):399–424.

56. Richiardi L, Bellocco R, Zugna D. Mediation analysis in epidemiology: methods, interpretation and bias. *Int J Epidemiol*. 2013;42(5):1511–1519.

57. Kim B. Introduction to mediation analysis. http://data.library.virginia.edu/introduction-to-mediation-analysis/.

58. Liu L, Nunez AE, Yu X, Yin X, Eisen HJ, for Urban Health Research G. Multilevel and spatial-time trend analyses of the prevalence of hypertension in a large urban city in the USA. *J Urban Health*. 2013;90(6):1053–1063.

59. Vermeulen E, Stronks K, Visser M, et al. Dietary pattern derived by reduced rank regression and depressive symptoms in a multi-ethnic population: the HELIUS study. *Eur J Clin Nutr*. 2017.

60. Briollais L, Durrieu G. Application of quantile regression to recent genetic and-omic studies. *Hum Genet*. 2014;133(8):951–966.

61. Liu L. Using multivariate quantile regression analysis to explore cardiovascular risk differences in subjects with chronic kidney disease by race and ethnicity: findings from the US chronic renal insufficiency cohort study. *Int Cardiovasc Forum J*. 2015;2(1).

CHAPTER 2

Pathophysiology and Risk Profiles of Heart Failure

THE PATHOPHYSIOLOGY OF HEART FAILURE

Heart failure is a serious condition. It happens when the heart cannot pump enough blood and oxygen to meet tissue metabolic requirements or support other organs in your body. Fig. 2.1 depicts the basic anatomy of the healthy heart and heart failure.[1]

Basic Concepts

Heart failure versus congestive heart failure

International Classification of Diseases, Tenth Revision, Clinical Modification (ICD-10-CM) codes heart failure as I50.1–I50.9, and *ICD-9-CM* as 428.0–428.0. It is a broad term in patients with the disorder. Table 2.1 shows the *ICD-9-CM* and *ICD-10-CM* for heart failure.[2,3]

Congestive heart failure is a type of heart failure and is the most severe clinical manifestation of heart failure. In patients with heart failure, his/her blood flow out of the heart becomes slowing, blood returning to the heart through the veins backs up, causing congestion in the body's tissues. Because not all patients have volume overload at the time of initial or subsequent evaluation, the term "heart failure" is preferred over the older term "congestive heart failure."[4]

The clinical syndrome of heart failure may result from disorders of the pericardium, myocardium, endocardium, and heart valves. Heart failure may also be associated with a broad spectrum of left ventricular (LV) functional abnormalities. It can range from patients with normal LV size and preserved ejection fraction to those with severe dilatation or reduced ejection fraction.

Ejection fraction (EF) is an important indicator in the classification of patients with heart failure; those who have heart failure with preserved ejection fraction are classified as heart failure with preserved ejection fraction (HFpEF), and those with reduced ejection fraction as heart failure with reduced ejection fraction (HFrEF). It is preferable to use these terms (HFpEF and HFrEF) over preserved or reduced systolic function.[5]

Pathophysiologic models of heart failure

Heart failure is a multisystem disorder characterized by abnormalities of cardiac function, skeletal muscle, renal function, stimulation of the sympathetic nervous system, and an intricate pattern of neurohormonal changes that impairs the ability of either ventricle to fill with or eject blood.[6,7] Over the past decades, three pathophysiologic models (hypotheses) for heart failure have been suggested.

Healthy heart

Heart failure

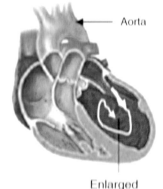

Aorta

Heart muscle pumps blood into the aorta in a healthy heart.

Left Ventricle

Aorta

Weakened heart Muscle cannot pump enough blood into the aorta. Blood pools in the heart, resulting in heart failure.

Enlarged heart

FIG. 2.1 The anatomy of healthy heart and heart failure. (From CDC Heart Failure, 2016.)

TABLE 2.1
International Classification of Diseases (ICD) 9 and 10 for Heart Failure

	ICD-9-CM		ICD-10-CM
ICD-9	**Description**	**ICD-10**	**Description**
428	Heart failure, code, if applicable heart failure due to hypertension first	**150**	Heart failure (HF). Code first: HF complicating abortion or ectopic or major pregnancy, HF following surgery, HF due to hypertension (HTN), HTN with chronic kidney disease, obstetric surgery and procedures, rheumatic HF
428.0	Congestive heart failure, unspecified	150.9	Heart failure, unspecified
428.1	Left heart failure	150.1	Left ventricular failure
428.20	Systolic heart failure, unspecified	150.20	Unspecified systolic (congestive) heart failure
428.21	Systolic heart failure, acute	150.21	Acute systolic (congestive) heart failure
428.22	Systolic heart failure, chronic	150.22	Chronic systolic (congestive) heart failure
428.23	Systolic heart failure, acute on chronic	150.23	Acute on chronic systolic (congestive) heart failure
428.30	Diastolic heart failure, unspecified	150.30	Unspecified diastolic heart failure
428.31	Diastolic heart failure, acute	150.31	Acute diastolic (congestive) heart failure
428.32	Diastolic heart failure, chronic	150.32	Chronic diastolic heart failure
428.33	Diastolic heart failure, acute on chronic	150.33	Acute on chronic diastolic heart failure
428.40	Combined systolic and diastolic heart failure, unspecified	150.40	Unspecified combined systolic and diastolic (congestive) heart failure
428.41	Combined systolic and diastolic heart failure, acute	150.41	Acute combined systolic and diastolic (congestive) heart failure
428.42	Combined systolic and diastolic heart failure, chronic	150.42	Chronic combined systolic and diastolic (congestive) heart failure
428.43	Combined systolic and diastolic heart failure, acute on chronic	150.43	Acute on chronic combined systolic and diastolic heart failure
428.9	Heart failure, unspecified	150.9	Heart failure, unspecified

- The cardiorenal model, in which heart failure is reviewed as a problem of excessive salt and water retention that is caused by abnormalities of renal blood flow.
- The cardiocirculatory, or hemodynamic, model, in which heart failure is thought to arise largely as a result of abnormalities in the pumping capacity of the heart and excessive peripheral vasoconstriction.
- The neurohormonal model, in which heart failure progresses as a result of the overexpression of biologically active molecules that are capable of exerting toxic effects on the heart and circulation.[8,9]

Classifications and Heart Failure Stages
NYHA functional classification
The New York Heart Association (NYHA) functional classification provides a simple way of classifying the extent of heart failure. It places patients in one of four categories based on how much they are limited during physical activity; the limitations and symptoms are regarding normal breathing and varying degrees in shortness of breath and/or angina.[10]

Class I: Cardiac disease, but no symptoms and no limitation in ordinary physical activity, e.g., no shortness of breath when walking and climbing stairs.

Class II: Mild symptoms (mild shortness of breath and/or angina) and slight limitation during ordinary activity.

Class III: Marked limitation in activity due to symptoms, even during less-than-ordinary activity, e.g., walking short distances (20–100 m) and/or being comfortable only at rest.

Class IV: Severe limitations. Experiences symptoms even while at rest and/or mostly bedbound patients.

TABLE 2.2			
The New York Heart Association (NYHA) Functional Classification and the American College of Cardiology/American Heart Association (ACC/AHA) Heart Failure Stages			
NYHA Functional Class		**ACC/AHA HF STAGES**	**Prevention and Treatment Strategies**
None	**A**	At high risk for developing hear failure, without structural heart disease or symptoms of HF	1. Adherence to healthy lifestyle modification (exercise, no smoking, weight control, and healthy food). 2. Treat comorbidities (e.g., hypertension, hyperlipidemia, diabetes, chronic kidney disease, or coronary artery disease).

I No limitation of physical activity	**B**	Structural heart disease but without symptoms of HF	1. Continue to treat comorbidities and adherence to healthy lifestyle.
			 2. Monitor for development of HF symptoms.
			 3. Additional treatment for reduced EF patients only:
			   i. Initiate β-blockers and ACE inhibitors or ARBs.
			   ii. Use implantable cardioverter defibrillators (ICDs) in post-MI patients.

II Slight limitation of physical activity
 	
 III Marked limitation of physical activity. (A small proportion of patients at NYHA Class III may belong to those in ACC/AHA Stage D)
	C	Structural heart disease but with prior or current symptom of HF	1. Continue to treat comorbidities and adherence to healthy lifestyle.
			 2. Educate patients on self-care (e.g., salt restriction) and HF symptoms.
			 3. Additional treatment for reduced EF patients only:
			   i. Initiate β-blockers and ACE inhibitors or ARBs with diuretics. Escalate pharmacologic treatment based on symptoms.
			   ii. Utilize ICDs or cardiac resynchronization therapy in post-MI patients.

IV Inability to carry on any physical activity	**D**	Refractory HF requiring specialized interventions	1. Refer to cardiology for advanced therapies, such as left ventricular assist device or heart transplant, when indicated. 2. Discuss end-of-life treatment goals, as appropriate.

ACE, angiotensin-converting enzyme; *ARB*, angiotensin receptor blocker; *EF*, ejection fraction; *HF*, heart failure, *MI*, myocardial infarction.

ACC and AHA heart failure staging

In 2001, the American College of Cardiology (ACC) and the American Heart Association (AHA) took a new approach to the classification of heart failure that emphasized both the evolution and progression of the disease. According to the ACC and AHA new approach, heart failure is identified as four stages.[11]

Stage A identifies the patient who is at high risk of developing heart failure but has no structural disorder of the heart.

Stage B refers to a patient with a structural disorder of the heart but who has never developed symptoms of heart failure.

Stage C denotes the patient with past or current symptoms of heart failure associated with underlying structural heart disease.

Stage D designates the patient with end-stage disease who requires specialized treatment strategies such as mechanical circulatory support, continuous inotropic infusions, cardiac transplantation, or hospice care.

The advantages and limitations of the NYHA functional classification of heart failure have been discussed in recent years.[12] Table 2.2 shows an overall comparison between the NYHA functional classification and the ACC/AHA stages of heart failure.[11,13,14]

Significance

The importance of classifying the subtypes HFrEF and HFpEF

The EF is an important measurement in determining how well the heart is pumping out blood and in diagnosing and tracking heart failure. Approximately half of all patients with heart failure have preserved ejection fraction (HFpEF), and they often include women and elderly. Thus, as life expectancies continue to increase in Western societies, the prevalence of HFpEF will continue to grow. Many features of the heart failure syndrome are similar across the EF spectrum, including elevated left atrial pressure, abnormal LV filling dynamics, neurohumoral activation, dyspnea, impaired exercise tolerance, frequent

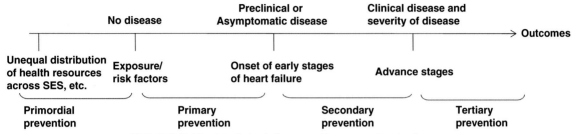

FIG. 2.2 Epidemiologic basis for preventive approaches to disease.

hospitalization, and reduced survival. In contrast to (classical) heart failure with reduced ejection fraction (HFrEF), only a limited spectrum of treatment modalities seem useful in improving morbidity and mortality rates in HFpEF.[15] Therefore, awareness and attention to the heart failure syndrome in the presence of normal or mildly abnormal EF are critical.

The importance of the ACC and AHA staging heart failure

The ACC/AHA classification system is intended to complement but not to replace the NYHA functional classification. It has been recognized for many years, however, that the NYHA functional classification reflects a subjective assessment by a physician and changes frequently over short periods and that the treatments used do not differ significantly across the classes. Therefore, the committee of ACC and AHA "believed that a staging system was needed that would reliably and objectively identify patients in the course of their disease and would be linked to treatments that were uniquely appropriate at each stage of their illness. According to this new approach, patients would be expected to advance from one stage to the next unless progression of the disease was slowed or stopped by treatment. This new classification scheme adds a useful dimension to our thinking about heart failure similar to that achieved by staging systems for other disorders."[11]

Fig. 2.2 depicts the epidemiologic basis for preventive approaches to disease. Traditionally, there were three levels of prevention (primary, secondary, and tertiary). The idea of "primordial prevention" was first introduced by Toma Strasser in 1978.[16] These four levels of preventions have been defined and applied in disease prevention and control.[16]

Primordial prevention

Primordial prevention, a relatively new concept, is defined as prevention of risk factors themselves, beginning with a change in social and environmental conditions known to increase the risk of disease. It aspires to establish and maintain conditions that minimize hazards to health. The primordial prevention is the task of public health policy and health promotion.[16]

Primary prevention

Primary prevention aims to reduce the incidence of disease, such as enhancing nutritional status, immunizing against communicable diseases, and eliminating environmental risks (such as contaminated drinking water supplies). The primary prevention is the task of health promotion, public health, and specific prevention.[16]

Secondary prevention

Secondary prevention aims to reduce the prevalence of disease by shortening its duration, such as by the use of screening a disease at an early stage. The secondary prevention is the task of presymptomatic diagnosis, treatment, and preventive medicine.[16]

Tertiary prevention

Tertiary prevention aims to soften the impact of long-term disease and disability by eliminating or reducing impairment, disability, and handicap; minimizing suffering; and maximizing potential years or useful like. The tertiary prevention is the task of treatment for late symptomatic disease and rehabilitation.[16]

Rehabilitation is the combined and coordinated use of medical, social, educational, and vocational measures for training and retraining patients to the highest possible level of functional ability. Recent studies suggest four types of rehabilitation: medical, social, vocational, and psychologic rehabilitations. Each type not only plays a unique role in rehabilitation treatment for a late symptomatic disease, but they also have multiple interactive effects on the results of the rehabilitation.

RISK FACTORS FOR HEART FAILURE
Basic Concepts

Several risk factors have been suggested to a causal role in the development of heart failure, although it remains the subject of debate. As heart failure is a syndrome rather than a primary diagnosis, it has many potential etiologies, diverse clinical features, and various clinical subsets. However, some patients may have a variety of major cardiovascular diseases, but never develop cardiac dysfunction, and others in whom cardiac dysfunction is identified through testing may never develop clinical heart failure. In addition to cardiac dysfunction, other factors, such as vascular stiffness, atrial dyssynchrony, and renal sodium handling, play significant roles in the manifestation of the syndrome of heart failure.[17]

Risk factors for heart failure

To highlight the differences in clinical treatment and prevention of heart failure, several approaches have been used to classify risk factors for heart failure according to their specific concerns. For example, the AHA proposes two groups of risks for heart failure.

- Lifestyle factors that increase the risk of heart disease, stroke, and diabetes (e.g., smoking, being overweight, and eating foods high in fat and cholesterol and physical inactivity).
- Health conditions that either damage the heart or make it work too hard. These conditions include (1) coronary heart disease (CHD); (2) past heart attack (myocardial infarction); (3) high blood pressure; (4) abnormal heart valves; (5) heart muscle disease (dilated cardiomyopathy, hypertrophic cardiomyopathy) or inflammation; (6) congenital heart disease; (7) severe lung disease, when the lungs do not work properly, the heart has to work harder to get available oxygen to the rest of the body; (8) diabetes; (9) obesity; (10) sleep apnea; and (11) others: low red blood cell count (severe anemia), hyperthyroidism, and arrhythmia.[18]

Schocken and Bui et al., according to the knowledge of the established and hypothesized risk factors, proposed eight groups of risk factors for heart failure.

- Major clinical risk factors: aging, males, hypertension, LV hypertrophy, myocardial infarction, valvular heart disease, obesity, and diabetes.
- Minor clinical risk factors: smoking, dyslipidemia, chronic kidney disease, albuminuria, sleep disordered breathing, anemia, increased heart rate, dietary risk factors, sedentary lifestyle, low socioeconomic status, and psychologic stress.
- Immune mediated risk factors: Peripartum cardiomyopathy and hypersensitivity.
- Infections: Viral, parasitic (Chagas disease), and bacterial.

- Toxic risk precipitants: Chemotherapy (anthracyclines, cyclophosphamide, 5-fluorouracil), targeted cancer therapy (trastuzumab, tyrosine kinase inhibitors), cocaine, nonsteroidal antiinflammatory drugs (NSAIDs), thiazolidinediones, doxazosin, and alcohol consumption.
- Genetic risk predictors: SNP (e.g., α2CDel322-325, β1Arg389), family history, and history of congenital heart disease.
- Morphologic risk predictors: Increased LV internal dimension, mass, and asymptomatic LV dysfunction.
- Biomarker risk predictors: Immune activation (e.g., insulin-like growth factors 1 [IGF1], tumor necrosis factor [TNF], interleukin 6 [IL-6], C-reactive protein [CRP]), natriuretic peptides (e.g., brain natriuretic peptide [BNP] and n-terminal [NT]-BNP), and high-sensitivity cardiac troponin.[19,20]

In the epidemiologic study and data analysis, we may classify risk factors for heart failure into five groups.

- Demographic factors: Age, sex, race/ethnicity, family history, including genetics.
- Lifestyle and behavior risk factors: Diet, smoking, physical activity, and alcohol consumption.
- Medical conditions: Hypertension, CHD, diabetes, chronic kidney disease, etc.
- Biomarkers: Manures of lipid profiles, metabolic disorder, inflammation, and electrocardiogram and echocardiogram, etc.
- Socioeconomic and environmental determinants.

The Complex Risk Factors and Outcomes Models of Heart Failure

Although a single risk factor may be enough to cause heart failure, its effect may come from an accumulative action and/or a combination effect of multivariable and multilevel risk factors on the risk of heart failure. Fig. 2.3 depicts an example of the conceptual model for major risk factors of heart failure and outcome study that is applied in our ongoing studies.

Impacts of Selected Risk Factors on Heart Failure

In epidemiologic studies, we can estimate their individual and combined (i.e., jointed) effects, including interaction effects on the risk of heart failure. To express these effects, we estimate the relative risk (RR), or odds ratios (OR), or hazard ratios (HR) of risk factors for heart failure. RR, OR, and HR have a similar meaning, but each comes from a study with an individual study design. For example, RR and HR are

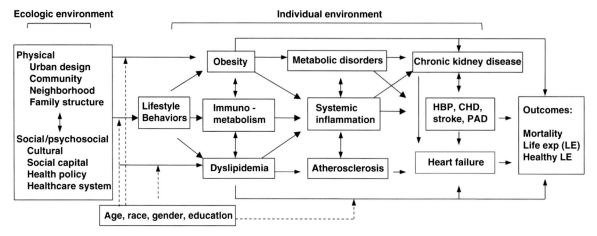

--- ▶ *Effect modification; HBP: hypertension; CHD: coronary heart disease; PAD: peripheral arterial disease; LE: life expectancy.*

FIG. 2.3 Risk factor model for heart failure and outcomes.

estimated in a prospective cohort study, and OR from studies with a cross-sectional or case-control study designs. The estimated RR (or OR, HR) of a risk factor (or combined) associated with the study outcomes of interest indicates a comparison between those with and without exposure to the risk factor of interest. Population attributable risk (PAR) is an estimate of incidence, prevalence, or mortality that would achieve if the population were entirely unexposed to the risk factor of interest. Table 2.3 shows some examples of factors associated with the risk of heart failure.[21–25] For example, in Dunlay and colleagues study, they reported that the odd of heart failure was 3.05 times higher (OR) in patients with CHD versus those without CHD. If CHD could be prevented, an estimate of 20% (PAR) of patients with heart failure would be reduced.[22] Individuals who were obese had 1.98 times

higher risk (HR) of having heart failure than those with a normal body mass index (BMI: 18.5–24.9 kg/m²).[21] More details of OR, RR, HR, and PAR will be discussed in Chapter 3.

Significance

Heart failure poses a serious clinical and public health issue. The lifetime risk of developing heart failure is one in five. Although cumulative evidence shows that the age-adjusted incidence of heart failure may have decreased or plateaued, heart failure is still one of the principal causes of morbidity and mortality, with 5-year mortality that rivals those of many cancers. Therefore, understanding of these risk factors for heart failure plays a pivotal role in the education of healthy lifestyle habits and in clinical practice for the purpose of control and prevention of this disease.

TABLE 2.3
Odds Ratios or Hazard Ratios of Risk Factors for Heart Failure

Risk Factors	Prevalence of HF OR	Incidence of HF HR	Mortality of HF HR	PAR	References
Coronary heart disease	3.05			0.20	Dunlay[22]
Diabetes	2.65			0.12	
Obese	2.00			0.12	
Hypertension	1.44			0.20	
Ever smoker	1.37			0.14	
BMI (REF: 18.5–24.9, KG/M^2)					
Overweight (18.5–24.9)		1.39			Kenchaiah[21]
Obese (>30)		1.98			
NUMBER OF PACK-YEARS OF CIGARETTE SMOKING					
1–11		1.13			Gopal[23]
12–35		1.35			
>35		1.64			
UNPROCESSED RED MEAT (G/D)					
<25.0		1			Kaluza[24]
25.0–49.9		1.14			
50.0–74.9		1.20			
>75.0 (83.5)		0.77			
PROCESSED RED MEAT (G/D)					
<25.0					
25.0–49.9		1.22			
50.0–74.9		1.42			
>75.0 (83.5)		2.43			
FOR ISCHEMIC HEART FAILURE					
Age (per year)			1.05		Zamora[25]
Left ventricular EF			0.98		
Diabetes			2.45		
Peripheral vascular disease			1.62		
β-blockers			0.28		
ACE-I/ARB			0.26		

ACE-I, angiotensin-converting enzyme inhibitor; *ARB*, angiotensin II receptor blocker; *EF*, ejection fraction; *HF*, heart failure; *OR*, odds ratios; *HR*, hazard ratios; *PAR*, population attributable risk.

REFERENCES

1. Centers for Disease Control and Prevention. Heart Failure. 2016; https://www.cdc.gov/dhdsp/data_statistics/fact_sheets/fs_heart_failure.htm. Accessed Nov 16, 2016.
2. American College of Cardiology. Heart failure: differences between ICD-10-CM and ICD-9-CM terminology. http://www.acc.org/tools-and-practice-support/practice-solutions/coding-and-reimbursement/icd-10/monthly-tips/icd10%20tips/december-heart-failure-differences-between-icd-10-and-icd-9-cm-terminology.
3. ICD-10 LifeLine for Physicians. Diagnosis: congestive heart failure. https://www.beaumont.edu/Global/Doctor/ICD10/icd-10_lifeline_for_physicians-feb.26.pdf.
4. Hunt SA, Abraham WT, Chin MH, et al. ACC/AHA 2005 Guideline Update for the Diagnosis and Management of Chronic Heart Failure in the Adult: a report of the American College of Cardiology/American Heart Association Task Force on Practice Guidelines (Writing Committee to Update the 2001 Guidelines for the Evaluation and Management of Heart Failure): developed in collaboration with the American College of Chest Physicians and the International Society for Heart and Lung Transplantation: endorsed by the Heart Rhythm Society. *Circulation.* 2005;112(12):e154–235.
5. Yancy CW, Jessup M, Bozkurt B, et al. ACCF/AHA guideline for the management of heart failure. *Circulation.* 2013. http://dx.doi.org/10.1161/CIR.0b013e31829e8776.
6. Jackson G, Gibbs CR, Davies MK, Lip GY. ABC of heart failure. Pathophysiology. *BMJ.* 2000;320(7228):167–170.
7. Mann DL. Mechanisms and models in heart failure: a combinatorial approach. *Circulation.* 1999;100(9):999–1008.
8. Batlle M, Perez-Villa F, Garcia-Pras E, et al. Down-regulation of matrix metalloproteinase-9 (MMP-9) expression in the myocardium of congestive heart failure patients. *Transpl Proc.* 2007;39(7):2344–2346.
9. Mann DL, Bristow MR. Mechanisms and models in heart failure: the biomechanical model and beyond. *Circulation.* 2005;111(21):2837–2849.
10. New York Heart Association. *The Criteria Committee of the New York Heart Association, Functional Capacity and Objective Assessment. Nomenclature and Criteria for Diagnosis of Diseases of the Heart and Great Vessels.* Boston, MA: Little Brown and Company; 1994:253–255.
11. Hunt SA, Baker DW, Chin MH, et al. ACC/AHA guidelines for the evaluation and management of chronic heart failure in the adult: executive summary: a report of the american college of cardiology/american heart association task force on practice guidelines (committee to revise the 1995 guidelines for the evaluation and management of heart failure) developed in collaboration with the international society for heart and lung transplantation endorsed by the heart failure society of america. *J Am Coll Cardiol.* 2001;38(7):2101–2113.
12. Raphael C, Briscoe C, Davies J, et al. Limitations of the New York Heart Association functional classification system and self-reported walking distances in chronic heart failure. *Heart.* 2007;93(4):476–482.
13. Committee NYHAC, Association NYH. *Nomenclature and Criteria for Diagnosis of Diseases of the Heart and Great Vessels.* Little, Brown Medical Division; 1979.
14. Farrell MH, Foody JM, Krumholz HM. β-Blockers in heart failure: clinical applications. *JAMA.* 2002;287(7):890–897.
15. Alonso-Betanzos A, Bolón-Canedo V, Heyndrickx GR, Kerkhof PL. Exploring guidelines for classification of major heart failure subtypes by using machine learning. *Clin Med Insights Cardiol.* 2015;9(suppl 1):57.
16. Last JM, Spasoff RA, Harris SS, Thuriaux MC. *A Dictionary of Epidemiology.* International Epidemiological Association, Inc.; 2001.
17. Heart Failure Society of America. Executive summary: HFSA 2010 comprehensive heart failure practice guideline. *J Card Fail.* 2010;16(6):475–539.
18. AHA heart failure. Causes of heart failure. http://www.heart.org/HEARTORG/Conditions/HeartFailure/CausesAndRisksForHeartFailure/Causes-and-Risks-for-Heart-Failure_UCM_002046_Article.jsp#.WN1wtul1q02.
19. Schocken DD, Benjamin EJ, Fonarow GC, et al. Prevention of heart failure: a scientific statement from the American Heart Association Councils on Epidemiology and Prevention, Clinical Cardiology, Cardiovascular Nursing, and High Blood Pressure Research; Quality of Care and Outcomes Research Interdisciplinary Working Group; and Functional Genomics and Translational Biology Interdisciplinary Working Group. *Circulation.* 2008;117(19):2544–2565.
20. Bui AL, Horwich TB, Fonarow GC. Epidemiology and risk profile of heart failure. *Nat Rev Cardiol.* 2011;8(1):30–41.
21. Levy D, Kenchaiah S, Larson MG, et al. Long-term trends in the incidence of and survival with heart failure. *N Engl J Med.* 2002;347(18):1397–1402.
22. Dunlay SM, Weston SA, Jacobsen SJ, Roger VL. Risk factors for heart failure: a population-based case-control study. *Am J Med.* 2009;122(11):1023–1028.
23. Gopal DM, Kalogeropoulos AP, Georgiopoulou VV, et al. Cigarette smoking exposure and heart failure risk in older adults: the Health, Aging, and Body Composition Study. *Am Heart J.* 2012;164(2):236–242.
24. Kaluza J, Åkesson A, Wolk A. Processed and unprocessed red meat consumption and risk of heart failure. A prospective study of men. *Circ Heart Fail.* 2014:6.
25. Zamora E, Lupón J, de Antonio M, et al. The obesity paradox in heart failure: is etiology a key factor? *Int J Cardiol.* 2013;166(3):601–605.

CHAPTER 3

Research and Design

CLINICAL EPIDEMIOLOGY AND TRANSLATIONAL EPIDEMIOLOGY

Basic Concepts

Clinical epidemiology

Clinical epidemiology is the application of the science of epidemiology in a clinical setting. Emphasis is on a medically defined population, as opposed to statistically formulated disease trends derived from examination of larger population categories. Overall, clinical epidemiology addresses patient-oriented outcomes and healthcare service research. For example, we conducted an intervention study (pilot) to improve adherence of the patients with heart failure to medication and healthy behaviors. In the study, we recruited 152 African American adults (males: 68, females: 84) who were diagnosed with heart failure. Of them, 79 were randomly assigned to the intervention group who received usual healthcare and cardiovascular health-focused intensive education and discussion through health-related survey questionnaires, and 73 participants who received usual healthcare for HF according to ACC/AHA guidelines and health-related questionnaire surveys. All patients received a baseline survey after their initial recruitment. All participants were invited to receive two times follow-up surveys by phone or in-person at hospital during their routinely scheduled healthcare visits. The first follow-up was conducted after 3 months and the second after an additional 3 months since the study assessment at baseline. The results show that the proportions of those with heart failure stages A, B, C, and D were 26.5%, 19.1%, 22.1%, and 10.3% in men, and 52.4%, 21.4%, 21.4%, and 4.8% in women, respectively. Of them, 121 completed the first (3 months), and 39 had both the first and second (3 months) follow ups. Significantly improved scores of knowledge to heart failure etiology and self efficacy were observed at the first follow up, and scores of self care skills were observed at the second follow up in both intervention and control groups. The improvement of knowledge to heart failure etiology and self efficacy healthcare scores in the intervention group were significantly higher in the first follow up ($P<.01$), and self care skill scores were higher in both the first and second follow ups ($P<.01$) than that in the control group. Significant improvement in adherence

to medication and healthy behaviors were observed in the intervention group ($P<.01$). There was a tendency of improvement in the quality of life in the periods of follow-up in the intervention group.[1]

The concepts of patient-oriented outcomes and healthcare service research in clinical epidemiology have been applied in clinical trials as well, for example, in the Antihypertensive and Lipid-Lowering Treatment to Prevent Heart Attack Trial, sponsored by the National Heart, Lung, and Blood Institute (NHLBI),[2] and in the Diabetes Prevention Program and Outcomes Study (DPPOS), sponsored by the National Institute of Diabetes and Digestive and Kidney Diseases (NIDDK) of the National Institutes of Health.[3]

In recent decades, advances in our understanding of human biology and the emergence of powerful new technologies, such as genomics and bioinformatics, provide us new insights into modern epidemiology. However, the transformation of scientific discoveries and advances into effective health interventions remains limited. Recent emphasis on translational research (TR) is highlighting the role of epidemiology in translating scientific discoveries into population health impact. For example, Khoury and his colleagues proposed the applications of epidemiology in TR through four phases (designed T1-T4), illustrated by examples from human genomics.[4] In T1, epidemiology explores the role of a new scientific discovery in applying in practice (such as a new biomarker used in risk prediction and prevention). In T2, epidemiology can help to evaluate the efficacy of a candidate application using observational studies and randomized controlled trials. In T3, epidemiology can help to assess facilitators and barriers for uptake and implementation of candidate applications in practice. In T4, epidemiology can contribute to assessing the impact of using candidate applications on population health outcomes. In the Ogilvie and colleagues study, they addressed two research gaps in population TR, the first between basic research and early clinical trials and the second between health technology assessment and healthcare delivery.[5]

Translational epidemiology

Translational epidemiology addresses the effective transfer of new knowledge from epidemiologic studies into the planning of population-wide and individual-level disease control programs and policies.[4,6,7] For example, the Heart Failure Association of the European Society of Cardiology recently organized an expert workshop to address the issue of inflammation in heart failure from basic science, translational and clinical perspective, and to assess whether specific inflammatory pathways may yet serve as novel therapeutic targets for this condition. In the workshop, several translational studies were reviewed and were consistent to address that chronic inflammation, interplaying with increased oxidative stress, cytokine production, proteolytic matrix degradation, and autoimmunity, is implicated in heart failure pathophysiology by increasing cardiac injury, fibrosis, and vascular dysfunction. One of the significant main findings is that "the idea of a common inflammatory pathway that characterizes all different forms of HEART FAILURE appears unrealistic. It will probably be important to design specific anti-inflammatory approaches for various types and stages of heart failure. In particular, anti-inflammatory approaches may need to differ markedly in acute vs. chronic HEART FAILURE."[6]

Significance

Clinical epidemiology addresses hospital-based study, and translational epidemiology addresses a whole aspect of basic, clinical, preventive, and predicting study. These basic concepts are fundamental in the study of heart failure epidemiology.

THE CREDIBILITY OF STUDY

The credulity criteria are involved in establishing that the results of a study are believable. It depends on the richness and accuracy of information gathered, rather than the amount of data collection. Two most common error factors affect the credibility of a study: (1) systematic error (bias) and (2) chance error (sampling variability).[8]

Bias

Bias is a systematic distortion of the association between a determinant (i.e., exposure) and an outcome due to a deficiency in the study design. It may arise (1) from the study sample that is not representative of the target population of interest (selection bias). (2) It is from incorrect use of instruments or from poor measurement (information bias), or (3) from the differential effects of other determinants on the association between exposures and outcomes of the interest (confounding).

Selection bias

Selection bias can occur from the study design and during the courses of the survey implementation. This bias may occur when the sample does not represent the target population of interest. For example, when some eligible participants refuse to participate in a study, the nonparticipation may introduce a selection bias. In particular, if the proportion of participants depends on both exposure and disease status, the estimate of association would be biased.

Information bias

Information bias refers to bias arising from measurement error. Information bias is known as observational bias and misclassification. For example, often, a variable can be measured by many different methods, and each method would have its accuracy. The most accurate method may be the most expensive, most time-consuming, or most invasive. This approach, however, may not be applied to all participants of a study population. In this case, another less expensive, less time-consuming, or less invasive method would be used to collect the information about the variable for all the participants. Certainly, an internal validation study is needed for obtaining information about the variable in a subsample of the study population from both the less accurate method and the more accurate method. The information about the variable would then be compared in the subsample. This comparison would yield values for the bias parameter (e.g., sensitivity and specificity) used to correct for classifying and correcting errors in the complete study population.[9]

Confounding

Confounding is one of the most intriguing biases that occur in an epidemiologic study. It arises whenever an outcome has multiple determinants (e.g., exposures), which are themselves associated, and one or more of them is omitted from the consideration in data collection and analysis. In epidemiologic studies, age and sex are most commonly treated as confounders because they are associated with exposures and are risk (or protective) factors for the outcomes of interest in most cases. For example, several studies demonstrate that decreased serum 25-hydrovitamin D concentration (a biomarker of vitamin D level in blood) is a risk factor for the development of heart failure and all-cause mortality.[10–14] Fig. 3.1 depicts that when we test whether decreased serum 25-hydrovitamin D concentration is a significant risk factor for heart failure, we should take into consideration of their association with age. Because it frequently reports that older adults have lower serum 25-hydroxyvitamin level than the younger adults. Aging is a significant risk factor for the development of heart failure.

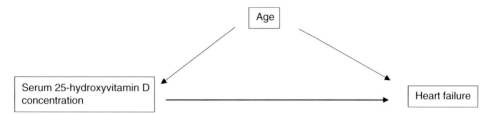

FIG. 3.1 A simple confounding case. To test whether there is an association between decreased serum 25-hydroxyvitamin D concentration (a biomarker for vitamin D intake) and risk of heart failure, we need to consider whether the association between serum 25-hydroxyvitamin D and heart failure, if any, is due to an association of age with serum 25-hydroxyvitamin D concentration and risk of heart failure. In the case, age is called a confounding factor and should be adjusted in the data analysis.

It is also well-recognized that serum 25-hydroxyvitamin D levels are different between males and females (e.g., females have higher serum 25-hydroxyvitamin D), and sex is a significant determinant of disease and mortality. Therefore, if our research of interest is to examine whether an exposure (instead of age and sex) is a predictor of disease, we need to control the effect of age and sex on the study of interest.

Definition of Confounder

A confounder is a variable that is associated with the exposure of interest and is a potential cause of the outcome of interest.

The characteristics of a potential confounder are as follows:
- It must be a risk factor for the outcome.
- It must be associated with the exposure of interest.
- It must not be an intermediate step in the causal pathway between the study exposure of interest and the outcome.
- It should not be a surrogate for exposure.

How can we control or decrease the potential confounding?

According to the steps of a study implementation, various ways could control or reduce the possibility of confounding across the three stages.
- Study design stage: Have an appropriate sample size and representative sample from the target population.
- Data collection stage: Follow a high quality of survey process and standard measures in data collection. Quality control and appropriate evaluation are always necessary to improve the quality of data.
- Data analysis stages: Stratification analysis, multivariate adjusted analysis (e.g., multivariate logistic regression), and sensitivity analysis can be applied to control potential confounding effects (see Chapters 4 and 5 for more detail).

ASSOCIATION, CAUSALITY, AND THE INTERPRETATION OF EPIDEMIOLOGIC EVIDENCE

One of the principal aims of an epidemiologic study is to assess the cause of disease whether the disease (or condition) occurs due to one or more risk factors (i.e., exposures). However, because most epidemiologic studies are by nature observational rather than experimental, several possible explanations for an observed association (either a statistically significant or nonsignificant association between an exposure and a disease) should be considered before we can infer that a cause-effect relationship exists. That is, an observed association may, in fact, be due to the effect of errors in over the course of the study design, implementation, and analysis. Therefore, an observed statistical association between a risk factor and a disease may not be necessarily a causal association. Conversely, the absence of an association does not necessarily imply the absence of a causal relationship.[15,16] To evaluate a statistical association, we need to examine three groups of errors.
- Chance (random error)
- Bias (systematic error)
- Confounding

A small sample size of a study may lead to low statistical power and be attributable to a nonsignificant statistical association between the study factors and the disease of interest. The nonsignificant finding may be caused, by chance, due to a small sample size. Estimating an appropriate sample size is critical in a study design.

Information and selection biases are two common errors in an observational study. Selection bias in participants' recruitment and information bias in data collection may cause systematic errors.

Non- or inappropriate adjustment analysis for confounders may cause serious confounding effects on the association between exposures and outcomes. For example, when we examine the association between diabetes and risk of heart failure, if we adjust for coronary heart disease, we may lead to an overadjustment because in most cases, coronary heart disease is on the pathway between diabetes and the risk of heart failure.

Even the above three groups of errors have been minimized or controlled appropriately; the judgment as to whether an observed statistical association (commonly defined as a *P*-value <.05, see Chapters 4 and 5) represents a cause-effect relationship between exposure and outcomes requires inferences far beyond the data from a single study. It involves consideration of criteria that include the magnitude of the association, the consistency of findings from other studies, and biologic credibility.[17]

The Bradford Hill criteria are widely used to assess whether an observed association is likely to be causal in an epidemiologic study.[18]

- The strength of the association between an exposure and an outcome: In general, the stronger the association between an exposure and an outcome, the more likely the relationship is to be causal. Relative risks (or odds ratios) are commonly used to assess the strength.
- The consistency of the findings by different studies: whether the same results are observed in different populations, in studies with different designs and different times.
- Specificity of the association between an exposure and an outcome: It must be a one-to-one relationship between a cause and an outcome.
- Temporal sequence of association: An exposure must precede an outcome.
- The biologic gradient between an exposure and an outcome: Change in disease rates should follow from corresponding changes in exposure, that whether

there is a dose-response relationship between the exposure levels and the severity of the disease.
- Biologic plausibility between an exposure and an outcome: Whether a potential biologic mechanism can explain this exposure-outcome relationship.
- Coherence with current knowledge: Does the relationship agree with the current understanding of the natural history or biology of the disease?
- Results from studies with experimental design: Does the removal of the exposure alter the frequency of the outcome?

EPIDEMIOLOGIC STUDY DESIGNS

Epidemiologic study design involves two main types of studies: descriptive and analytical studies. As discussed in Chapter 2, descriptive epidemiologic studies are concerned with describing the distribution of disease and risk factors by frequency concerning person, place, and time. Analytical epidemiologic studies are concerned with the causality of disease based on a comparison of study populations in related to their disease or exposure to risk factors' status. In general, to study the causes of disease, descriptive studies raise questions and provide the opportunity to generate hypotheses of the presence of an association between disease and exposures; and analytical studies test the hypotheses. There are two major descriptive epidemiologic study designs (i.e., ecologic study and cross-sectional study) and two major analytical epidemiologic study designs (i.e., observational studies and experimental studies). Fig. 3.2 depicts the two main types of epidemiologic study designs.

1) **Descriptive epidemiology** (person, place, and time)
    observational studies — describing burden of disease and generating research hypothesis:

    - Ecologic study (correlation study)
    - Cross-sectional study (prevalence study)

2) **Analytical epidemiology** (causal)
    examining risk of disease and testing research hypothesis

    - Observational studies — natural course of events
        Case-control study (regular and nested)
        Cohort studies (prospective and retrospective studies)

    - Experimental studies — investigator allocates exposure and follows subjects
        Randomized clinical trial (RCT)
        Community trial

FIG. 3.2 Two main types of epidemiologic study designs.

Ecologic Study

An ecologic study is also called as correlation study. The units of observations are usually geographically defined populations (e.g., not specific individuals) to describe disease frequencies between different groups during the same period or in the same population at various points in time about a presumed risk factor.

The advantage of the study is that it can be conducted relatively quick and at low cost because the requested data are relatively easy to obtain. The study is useful for the detection of research questions and the formulation of hypotheses for further research.

An ecologic study cannot be used to test a research hypothesis because of limitations inherent in this design. First, the lack of individual-level information leads to a limitation, known as the "ecologic fallacy" or "ecologic bias." The ecologic fallacy means that any association observed between variables on an aggregated level cannot be applied to the individual. An additional limitation of an ecologic study is that investigators are unable to detect subtle or complicated relationships between disease and exposures. It is because of the nature of the study design and character of the data collected. Data from an ecologic study lack information on the individuals' characteristics that might affect the association. Fig. 3.3 shows an example of an ecologic relationship between county-level age-adjusted prevalence of diabetes in 2013 and age-adjusted mortality of heart failure in 2013–2015 among US male adults aged 35 and older. It depicts that counties with higher rates of diabetes have higher mortality from heart failure compared with their counterparts. Although it raises a further research question on the association between these two diseases, it is not necessarily to interpret there is a casual relationship from the data.

To conduct an ecologic study, we should keep in mind:

- Because the units of observations are in groups either by geographic areas such as neighborhood, county, or state level prevalence of disease in the same study periods, or different points in time in the same populations, it is very likely their age distributions are different across the study areas or various points in time. Therefore, we should consider the differences. Age-standardization approaches for comparison between rates and means in an ecologic study are commonly requested before performing a correlation analysis.
- Sample size from each area or point in time should be big enough to have a representative rate or mean.
- Temporal issues between the study exposures and outcomes of interest should be considered. For example, although data for the exposure and outcome can be in the same period(s), or an earlier point in time for exposure variable than the outcome of interest, an exposure cannot be later than the outcome.

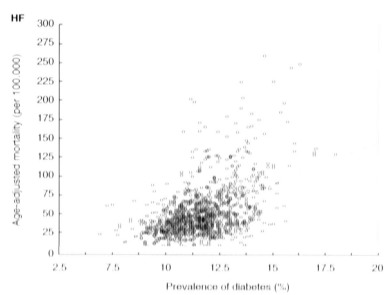

FIG. 3.3 Ecologic study: age-adjusted prevalence of diabetes (percentage) and mortality of heart failure (per 100,000 population) among male adults in US counties.

Cross-Sectional Study

A cross-sectional study describes the pattern of health-related events/factors and examines the relationship between disease and various risk or protective factors of interests in a defined population at one point in time.

Cross-sectional studies are carried out for public health planning and primary etiologic research. Most national health surveys conducted by the US National Center for Health Statistics are cross-sectional studies, for example, the National Hospital Discharge Surveys (NHDS), Nationwide Inpatients Sample, and Behavioral Risk Factor Surveillance Systems.[19–22]

Example

A cross-sectional study (n = 3000) aimed to describe the frequencies of diabetes and heart failure and to examine whether patients with diabetes have an increased risk of heart failure in a population aged 45 and older (Table 3.1). In the study, of the subjects (n = 2411) with diabetes mellitus (DM), the prevalence of heart failure was 16.83% [= a/(a + b) = 70/416], and among those without DM (n = 2584) the prevalence of heart failure was 5.53% [= c/(c + d) = 143/2584] (see Table 3.1). The results suggest that patients with DM had a higher rate of heart failure than those without DM. In statistics, for the type of Table 3.1, we call it a 2 × 2 table (or 2-by-2 table), showing four cells: a, b, c, and d, as given in Table 3.2. It is a primary table when we discuss how to test whether these two rates are statistically significant using chi-square test (see Chapter 4).

Successive cross-sectional studies can be used to examine if there are trends in disease and exposures over time (e.g., changes in prevalence of disease, exposure, or the strength of an association between disease and exposures over time). For example, using data from the NHDS, we examined the trend in the prevalence of hypertensive disease (HTD) and subtypes of HTD attributable to hospitalization among US adults aged 35 years and older from 1980 to 2007. We defined the primary cause of hospitalization for patients with the first-listed diagnosis of HTD and a comorbid condition of HTD for those who had any of the second- to seventh-listed diagnosis. Age-adjusted rates of disease were calculated using US 2000 standard population. The results show that age-adjusted hospitalization rates due to first diagnosis of HTD increased from 1.74% in 1980–1981 to 2.06% in 2006–2007 in men (P < .01) and from 2.0% to 2.09% in women (P = .06). Age-adjusted rates due to any of the second to the seventh diagnosis of HTD significantly increased from 7.06% to 35.09% in men (P < .001) and from 7.88% to 31.98% (P < .001) in women. Patients with the second to the seventh diagnosis of essential

TABLE 3.1
Number of Comorbidity Status

		HF Yes	HF No	Total
DM	Yes	70	346	416
		(a)	(b)	
	No	143	2441	2584
		(c)	(d)	
		213	2787	3000

DM, diabetes mellitus; HF, heart failure.

TABLE 3.2
Type of 2 × 2 Table

Exposure (Factor)	DISEASE Positive	DISEASE Negative	Total
Positive	a	b	a + b
Negative	c	d	c + d
Total	a + c	b + d	a + b + c + d

hypertension and hypertensive chronic kidney disease had the highest annual percent increases.[23]

Unlike an ecologic study, *cross-sectional studies* assess the status of participants on the presence or absence of the disease and exposure at the same point in time. Note that in this type of study, the cases of disease we identify are the prevalence of cases. We know that these cases have existed at the point in time of the study, but we commonly do not know their exact duration (i.e., a patient can be a newly diagnosed case or a previously diagnosed case). For this reason, a cross-sectional study is also called a *prevalence study*. Cross-sectional studies are routinely conducted to describe the burdens of disease and risk factors in population-based health surveys. Beyond the nature of the study design, if we have multiyears' serial cross-sectional data, we may examine potential cohort effects of different periods (such as changes in the environment and health policy by time) on the changes in risk of disease.[24,25] For example, Table 3.3 shows the prevalence rate (per 1000) of hospitalization in patients with the first-listed diagnosis of heart failure among males aged 35 and older, who participated in the US NHDS from 1980 to 2010.

Table 3.3 illustrates the relationship between data from calendar years and links with birth cohorts, for example, in a 1980 survey, patients aged 45–49 were born in 1931–35 (red). After 5 years (in a 1985 survey), the groups of participants (note: they were not the

TABLE 3.3
Prevalence (per 1000) of Hospitalization in Male Patients With Heart Failure

Age (years)	NHDS 1980–2010							Birth Cohort
	1980–84	1985–89	1990–94	1995–99	2000–04	2005–09	2010	
35–39	2.1	3.0	5.0	6.6	9.6	13.8	19.6	1971–75
40–44	2.7	6.3	8.4	10.7	13.5	17.1	11.9	1966–70
45–49	5.1	10.5	12.1	15.8	21.1	22.1	18.3	1961–65
50–54	6.8	13.5	20.4	24.0	26.7	29.1	26.8	1956–60
55–59	11.5	19.0	27.8	31.4	35.7	34.3	28.5	1951–55
60–64	15.5	26.3	37.1	37.9	42.1	39.1	40.3	1946–50
65–69	22.5	33.6	46.8	47.1	47.4	44.3	41.4	1941–45
70–74	31.8	44.4	55.4	56.2	54.1	50.0	45.3	1936–40
75–79	38.9	52.7	66.1	62.3	62.6	56.5	58.7	1931–35
>80	52.3	65.9	81.3	76.7	75.9	74.3	72.6	1926–30

NHDS, National Hospital Discharge Surveys.

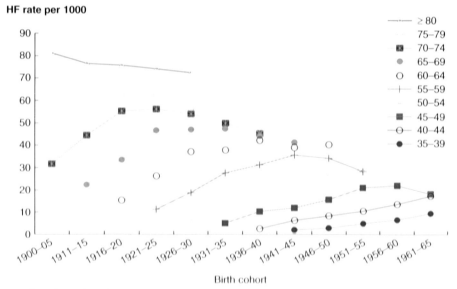

FIG. 3.4 Prevalence (per 1000) of hospitalization in patients with the first-listed diagnosis of heart failure (HF) by birth cohort in male adults, US NHDS 1980–2010.

same participants rather representing the same cohort of populations) were 5 years older (in the age group of 50–54 years). We then present the data in a birth cohort format shown in Fig. 3.4. It adds to evidence that there are increased trends of hospitalization in younger patients with heart failure among those who were born in recent decades. For example, the rate was 5.1% in patients aged 45–49 who were born in 1931–1935 (in

1980–1984 surveys). However, this rate increased to 22.1% in the same age group for those who were born in 1956–1960 (in 2005–2009 surveys).

Strengths of a cross-sectional study:
- Being quick and low cost
- Providing information on prevalence of disease and exposures
- Raising questions for further studies

- Providing evidence of birth cohort effects on changes in prevalence and mortality in multiple years
- Providing data from which hypotheses are generated
  Limitations of a cross-sectional study:
- Cannot establish cause-effect relationships. Because a disease determinant can change with time, a cross-sectional study can give misleading results. For example, a patient who smoked for years may quit smoking after he/she had a diagnosis of heart disease. If a cross-sectional study were conducted after the patient has quit smoking, he/she would be classified as those who are not currently smoking. In the case, we may find a weak association between current smoking and risk of disease because, in the comparison group, those who smoked before and are not currently smoking are included. Bias due to the survey design from a prevalence study is called prevalence bias.
- In a cross-sectional study, survival bias may exist as well. It occurs because some patients with severe disease status may have died after diagnosis or who recovered quickly are less likely to be identified in the prevalent patient group. Therefore, the patients who are "survivors" may be very different from those who die or recover quickly from the disease.

As discussed above, a cause-effect relationship of a disease determinant and the severity of the association between disease and risk factors may be underestimated in a cross-sectional study. To resolve this issue, a prospective cohort study that compares the incidence of a disease between those with and without exposure to the risk factors of interest over a period of follow-up is needed.

Prospective Study

A prospective study, or a prospective cohort study, is a longitudinal study in which participants are selected before they have experienced the outcomes of interest. Their exposures to possible determinants of interest are examined and recorded, together with their subsequent disease outcomes. In other words, a prospective cohort study is designed to compare disease incidence and/or mortality in populations classified by the condition whether the participants are exposed to the determinant(s) of interest or not. Fig 3.5 depicts the basic research process.

For example, let us set up a prospective cohort study to examine whether serum vitamin D insufficiency is a predictor for the risk of the development of heart failure. We can select a group of individuals who have lower serum 25-hydroxyvitamin D levels [25(OH)D, a marker of vitamin D intake] and a group of participants who have higher serum 25(OH)D levels. Both groups are free of heart failure at the beginning of the study. We record the numbers in each group who develop heart failure during a specified follow-up period (say, 10 years). Then we compare the incidence of heart failure between the two groups who are exposed to the lower or higher serum 25(OH)D levels (such as <20 ng/mL vs. >=20 ng/mL). If the incidence rates of heart failure are different between the two groups, and if the two groups are similar in every aspect except their exposure to the levels of serum 25(OH)D, we may conclude that the difference in the incidence of heart failure between the two groups is due to the risk factor alone.

Strengths of a prospective study:
- Compared with a cross-sectional study, a study with prospective cohort design may test a cause-effect association between exposures and outcomes because it is designed such that the determinants of interest occur before the development of the outcomes.
- Compared with a case-control study (see the next section), a cohort study minimizes selection bias and information bias because the participants are free of the outcomes of interest at the starting point of the study. Information on the determinants of interest is measured over the follow-up period, instead of recalling.

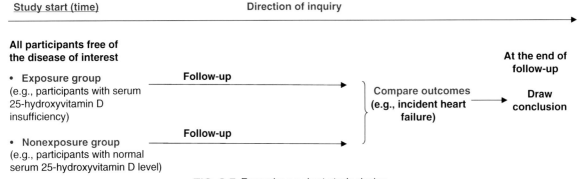

FIG. 3.5 Example: a cohort study design.

- A cohort study allows investigators to examine multiple outcomes.

Limitations of a prospective study:

- In general, a cohort study is very expensive because it may take years for the participants who develop the disease of interest.
- A cohort study is time-consuming because the development of a disease or an outcome of interest may take years to occur with a long period of follow-up.
- Exposures to risk factors may change over time.
- Inefficient for rare outcomes.
- Only a few possible determinants of the outcomes of interest could be examined due to the nature of the study design. It is evident that, if we missed measures of a few key covariates, we may reach a misleading conclusion. For example, in the sample study of serum 25(OH)D and risk of heart failure, if unknown to us, most of those who have higher serum vitamin D concentration are nonsmokers and most of those who have lower serum vitamin D concentration are smokers. Given that smoking is a well-established risk factor for heart failure, the association between subjects with lower serum vitamin D levels and those with a higher risk of the development of heart failure could be entirely due to the smoking factor. Therefore, a comparable approach to study designs (and data analysis) is critical in a cohort study (and any other types of epidemiologic comparison studies).
- The loss to follow-up is another issue in a cohort study. Some participants leave the geographic area of the study and cannot be traced; some die of unknown cause or lose interest to participate in the study continuously; some are inevitably "lost" to follow-up for any reasons, despite intensive efforts to track them. All these will introduce selection bias.

Retrospective cohort study

A major problem with a prospective cohort study design is that the study population often must be followed up for a period to determine whether the outcome of interest has developed. For example, in the study of the relationship between serum 25(OH)D concentration and risk of the development of heart failure, the study starts by selecting two groups: one has a lower 25(OH)D level and the other with normal serum 25(OH)D concentration. Both groups will be followed for several years, to see which group has a higher incidence of heart failure. This type of study design is called a *prospective cohort study* (or a longitudinal study). It is time consuming and costly. Given these issues, the prospective cohort study is often unattractive to investigators.

However, if the exposure of interest was well recorded for a long time in the past (such as serum 25(OH)D was measured several years ago), a *retrospective cohort study* can be designed. In a retrospective cohort study, both the exposures and outcomes have already occurred when the study begins. The study involves assembling the existing information on the persons' exposure status from the historical data and combining these data with the persons' outcome status. It is absolutely one can conduct a retrospective cohort study in a short period. For example, if we have a well-established electronic health record (EHR) system with several measures of interest are ready, a retrospective cohort study is feasible.

Steps to conduct a cohort study
- Define and measure exposure and identify nonexposed populations
- Follow-up (retrospective or prospective cohort study)
- Assessments of outcome
- Data analyses and interpretation

Example 1
To examine associations of unprocessed and processed red meat consumption (i.e., define exposures) with heart failure incidence and mortality (i.e., outcomes) in men, a population-based prospective Cohort of Swedish Men (COSM) study was conducted in 37,035 men aged 45–79 who had no history of heart failure, ischemic heart disease, or cancer at baseline (i.e., the study design and inclusion criteria). Within a mean follow-up of 11.8 years, 2891 incidences and 266 deaths resulted from heart failure. In the study, unprocessed and processed red meat consumption were categorized into four groups (<25, 25–49.9, 50–74.9, and ≥75 g/day) (i.e., define the exposure group). The results indicate that men who consumed ≥75 g/day processed red meat had 1.28 (95% confidence interval [CI]: 1.10–1.48) times higher risk of incident heart failure and 2.43 (95%CI: 1.52–3.88) times higher risk of death from heart failure compared with those who consumed <25 g/day.[25]

Example 2
A retrospective cohort study was conducted using data from the US Medicare beneficiaries and reports by Dr. Lindenauer and colleagues. Patients aged 65 years and older and hospitalized in 2006–08 with a principal diagnosis of acute myocardial infarction, heart failure, or pneumonia were examined the association between exposure to income inequality and patient's

risk of death or readmission within 30 days of a previous admission to an acute care hospital. *International Classification of Diseases, Ninth Revision* (*ICD-9*) was applied to identify the study disease of interest and mortality. The results show that there are 555,962 admissions in 4348 hospitals for acute myocardial infarction that met criteria for the 30-day mortality analysis, 1092,285 in 4484 hospitals for heart failure, and 1,146,414 in 4520 hospitals for pneumonia. The readmission analysis included 553,073 patients in 4262 hospitals for acute myocardial infarction, 1,345,909 hospitalizations in 4494 hospitals for heart failure, and 1,345,909 hospitalizations in 4524 hospitals for pneumonia. Results from the multilevel regression analysis indicate that there was no significant association between income inequality and mortality within 30 days of admission for patients with acute myocardial infarction, heart failure, or pneumonia. However, income inequality was significantly associated with rehospitalization in patients with acute myocardial infarction (risk ratio 1.09, 95%CI: 1.03–1.15), heart failure 1.07 (1.01–1.12), and pneumonia 1.09 (1.03–1.15).[26]

Case-Control Study

Compared with a cohort study, a case-control study may overcome some of these limitations and difficulties because it differs from a cohort study on the selection of participants. In a case-control study, patients who already have a disease (*case group*) and people who do not have the disease (*control group*) are selected. The proportions of each group with the exposures of interest are compared and tested.

Steps to conduct a case-control study
Selection of cases. Incident or prevalent cases are the cases selected from a hospital (or several hospitals), physicians' office, or patient registry.

Selection of controls. Nonhospitalized persons who do not have the disease:
- Community population
- Neighborhood
- Family member
- Patients without the disease of interest as controls

Data collection of past exposures to the risk factor(s) under study
Data collection should focus on the key elements of the study interest, including the exposure factors, covariates, and outcomes.

Data analyses and interpretation
Several common steps and approaches are discussed below.

Univariate analysis. Step 1: Calculate and describe the proportions, rates, means of the exposure factors, and key covariates, and then present them by case and control groups. The results may be named and presented as "the characteristics of cases and controls."

Step 2: Calculate odds ratios (OR), including OR 95%CI.

Multivariate analysis. In a case-control study, a logistic regression model is commonly used to analyze the dataset. Outcomes (binary or polynomial) are the dependent variable(s), and the exposures of the study interest are the independent variables. Covariates are the possible confounders to be adjusted.

Step 3 (continued from univariate analysis): It is better to adjust covariates individually or a set of small group step by step (e.g., demographic factors, socioeconomic-related factors, or behavioral factors as a group), instead of entering all covariates into a multivariate-adjusted model at the beginning, as we can evaluate the individual impact of a factor or a set of relevant factors on the outcome of interest.

Step 4: Fit final multivariate-adjusted model(s). In the step, you may apply stepwise procedures in logistic regression modeling or apply force-entry approach; it largely depends on the objectives of the study design and research questions.

Fig. 3.6 shows an overall process of conducting a case-control study.

Strengths of a case-control study
- Compared with a cohort study, a case-control study is relatively quick and inexpensive.
- It is a practical study design for investigating risk factors for rare disease.
- A case-control study can evaluate multiple risk factors for one disease because the study begins with individuals who already have the disease of interest and then collect data through recall history of their experience.

Limitations of a case-control study
- Selection bias is one of the main limitations in a case-control study because the selected cases have already had the disease of interest when the study begins, and the control are selected from a matching approach that depends on the availability at the point in time of the study.

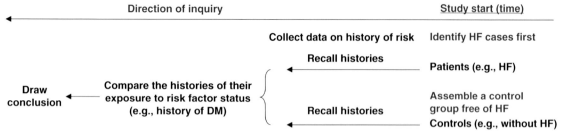

FIG. 3.6 Example: a case-control study design. *DM*, diabetes mellitus; *HF*, heart failure.

- In a case-control study, information on determinants (e.g., exposures) is obtained through participants' recall or their historically documented measures. Potential information bias (i.e., recall bias) may occur.
- It can only study one disease at a time.

Methods to improve the quality of a case-control study

Matching. Matching: For each case, find a control that looks just like him/her in all other possible ways except for the disease (e.g., matching on age, sex, and race).

- **Individual matching (one-to-one matching):** One case is matched to one control. For example, a case-control study aims to test whether drug A is a risk factor for heart failure. From the literature review, age is a probable confounding variable. Therefore, cases and controls should be matched by age, such as each 65-year-old patient with heart failure (case) will be matched with a healthy 65-year-old "control" person.
- **Frequency matching:** Rather than matching control to one patient, frequency matching requires that the frequency distributions of the matched variables be similar in case and control groups. For example, in a study, if the case group has 100 young men, 50 old men, 25 young women, and 25 old women, then the control group will be made the same. Frequency matching does not have to seek groups of equal sizes.

Multiple controls (one case matched to several controls): For each case, find one or more controls that are recommended by many epidemiologists when the number of controls is available (but there is little gain from having more than four matched controls per case).

Blinding: If it is possible, investigators who assess exposures should be blinded to whether the study subject is a case or control.

Case-control study versus cross-sectional study

- In a case-control study, subjects are samples from two populations (cases and controls), and cases may be incident or prevalent.
- In a cross-sectional study, subjects are sampled from one population, and cases are prevalent.

Example

In a report by Drs. Dunlay and colleagues, a case-control study was conducted to examine risk factors for heart failure. Residents living in Olmsted County, Minnesota, who had a new diagnosis of heart failure, identified by *ICD-9* code 428, between 1979 and 2002 were selected, and age- (±3 years older) and sex-matched population-based controls using Rochester Epidemiology Project resource were selected. The evidence for each risk factor of heart failure (i.e., coronary heart disease, hypertension, diabetes, obesity, smoking) was collected from age 18 until the date of incident heart failure or index date for controls. The results suggest that hypertension was the most common risk factor (population attributable risk, PAR = 66%), followed by smoking (51%). The risk of heart failure was particularly high for coronary heart disease and diabetes with OR (95%CI) of 3.03 (2.36–3.95) and 2.65 (1.98–3.54), respectively.[27]

Nested case-control study

A study design that has been used increasingly in recent years is the *nested case-control study*—a hybrid design in which a case-control study is nested in a cohort study. The cohort, at its inception or during follow-up, has had exposure information or biospecimens collected. The investigator identifies cases of disease that occurred in the cohort during the follow-up period. They also identify disease-free individuals within the cohort to serve as controls. Using previously collected data and obtaining additional measurements of exposures from available biospecimens, the investigator compares the exposure frequencies in cases and controls as in a non-nested case-control study.[28]

This design is shown schematically in Fig. 3.7.

Advantages of a nested case-control study
- Compared with a cohort study, a nested case-control study saves time and inexpensive.
- It has no or limited recall biases compared with a traditional case-control study.
- It is able to obtain incident data.
- It is able to examine a temporal relationship between exposures and outcomes.

Example
Drs. Hsiao and Hsieh et al. examined the association between the use of dopamine agonists and the risk of heart failure using a nested case-control study using data from Taiwan's National Health Insurance Research Database (NHIRD). They identified a population-based cohort comprising 27,135 patients who were prescribed antiparkinsonian drugs between 2001 and 2010. Of the patients, a nested case-control study was carried out in which 1707 cases of newly diagnosed heart failure were matched to 3414 controls (1:2 matched according to age, gender, and cohort entry year) within this cohort. Their results showed that an increased risk of heart failure was observed with the current use of ergot-derived dopamine agonists (adjusted OR 1.46, 95%CI: 0.997–2.12) but not with the current use of non–ergot-derived dopamine agonists (adjusted OR 1.24, 95%CI 0.84–1.82). Among non–ergot-derived dopamine agonists, both pramipexole (adjusted OR 1.40, 95%CI 0.75–2.61) and ropinirole (adjusted OR 1.22, 95%CI 0.76–1.95) showed a nonsignificantly increased heart failure risk. Although this study may be limited by the lack of statistical power, a clear pattern of an increased risk of heart failure was observed during the use of pramipexole.[29]

Experimental Studies
As distinct from an observational study (i.e., a cross-sectional, cohort, and case-control study), an experimental study is that the investigators have some control over a determinant of interest. From the study design, experimental studies are necessarily prospective (cohort) studies. A case-control study, however, cannot be experimental because the participants are selected after they have already been exposed to the determinant of interest.

Experimental studies are most commonly the studies that investigate treatment therapies for a disease of interest among patients or subjects with high risk of disease. Two major types of experimental studies (i.e., randomized trails) may be identified: (1) randomized clinical trials (i.e., where treatments and interventions are allocated to individuals at clinical settings) and (2) community trials (i.e., where treatments and/or interventions are assigned to entire communities).[16,30,31]

Designing an experimental study
Before a clinical or community trial begins, investigators review prior information about the intervention (such as a drug) to develop specific research questions and objectives. Although different studies have their specific research questions and objectives, investigators should keep in mind of two important aspects when generating research questions and objectives: (1) significance and (2) innovation.[32]

Significance: What are the significances of the study? Does the study address an important problem

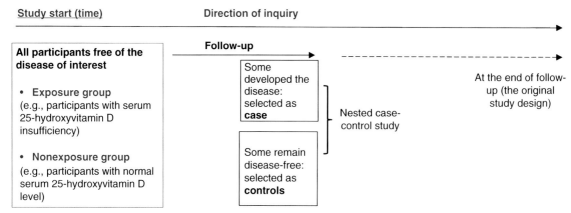

FIG. 3.7 Example: a nested case-control study design.

or a critical barrier to progress in the field? Is there a true scientific premise for the study? If the objectives of the study are achieved, how will scientific knowledge, technical capability, and/or clinical practice be improved? How will successful completion of the goals change the concepts, methods, technologies, treatments, services, or preventative interventions that drive this field?

Innovation: Does the study challenge and seek to shift current research or clinical practice paradigms by utilizing novel theoretical concepts, approaches or methodologies, instrumentation, or interventions? Are the concepts, approaches or methodologies, instrumentation, or interventions novel to one field of research or novel in a broad sense? Is a refinement, improvement, or new application of theoretical concepts, approaches or methodologies, instrumentation, or interventions proposed?

When specific research questions have been developed, then the investigators need to decide:
- Who qualifies to participate (selection criteria)?
- How many people will be part of the study?
- How long will the study last?
- Whether there will be a control group and other ways to limit research bias?
- How will the drug be given to patients and at what dosage?
- What assessments will be conducted, when, and what data will be collected?
- How will the data be reviewed and analyzed?

Fig. 3.8 shows the basic design of a randomized trial. We begin with a defined population that is randomized to receive either a new treatment or current treatment. We follow the subjects in each group to see how many are improved in the new treatment group compared with the current treatment group.

In a clinical trial, randomized controlled trial and double blinding are critical approaches to control potential confounding effects.

Randomized controlled trial: A method where the study population is divided randomly to mitigate the chances of self-selection by participants or bias by the study designers. Before an experiment begins, the investigators will assign the members of the participant pool to their groups (control, intervention, parallel).

Two methods are frequently applied in a randomization process:
- Using a random number table, which is created by statisticians and can be found in most biostatistics textbooks
- Computing assignment, most software can generate a random number and help the random assignments of case and control groups.

Some basic concepts in randomization trials
- Blinding: Subjects do not know which group they are assigned to in a study (single blind). It avoids certain psychologic responses that may affect the study if the study subject knows that he or she is receiving a new therapy or a placebo or usual care.
- Double blinding: Not only subjects do not know which group they are assigned to, but the data collectors (often including the physician) and data analysts are also blinded.
- Placebo: An inert substance that looks, tastes, and smells like the active agent (i.e., the new drug).

For example, a randomized controlled trial was conducted to evaluate the efficacy and safety of treatment with sildenafil (ClinicalTrials.gov number NCT00309790) for 12 weeks in patients with systolic heart failure receiving standard heart failure therapy.[11]

Study design
In the trial, placebo-controlled, double-blind, and parallel assignment methods were used to compare two groups of patients. One group received sildenafil and the other group received a placebo (a pill that looks like sildenafil but contains no medication). Patients had a heart catheterization, echocardiogram, and exercise stress test. Patients then took study medication for 12 weeks. A repeat heart catheterization, echocardiogram, and exercise stress test were then performed.

The inclusion and exclusion criteria of participants
The inclusion criteria for participants were (1) patients aged 18 years and older who had left ventricular (LV) systolic dysfunction (LV ejection fraction <40%), (2)

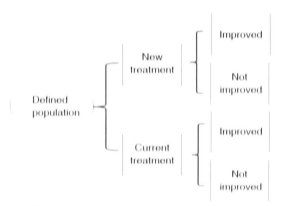

FIG. 3.8 The basic design of a randomized trial.

patients who had New York Heart Association class II–IV chronic heart failure, and (3) patients who had secondary pulmonary hypertension (PH, defined by a mean pulmonary arterial pressure >25 mm Hg). The exclusion criteria for participants were (1) patients who were taking the following medications: nitroglycerine pill/patch/paste, Isordil, Imdur, antifungal agents, and certain antidepressants; (2) patients who had a history of optic neuropathy or unexplained visual impairment, and/or with anemia.

Assignments and outcome measures

The primary outcome measures included (1) patients who had the following performed at baseline and again after taking sildenafil for 12 weeks: exercise capacity measured by exercise stress test and heart pressure measured by a heart catheterization; (2) the quality of life measured by the Minnesota Living With Heart Failure questionnaire at baseline and week 12 of the follow-up. A total of 37 patients who met the recruitment criteria were randomized to treatment and placebo groups for a 12-week trial.

Results

The results show that sildenafil improves exercise capacity and quality of life in patients with systolic heart failure and secondary PH. The change in peak V_{O2} from baseline, the primary end point, was greater in the sildenafil group (1.8 ± 0.7 mL/ kg min) than in the placebo group (−0.27 mL/kg min, $P = .02$).[34]

Clinical trial in drug development

In a new drug development, however, the U.S. Food and Drug Administration (FDA) describes a clinical trial with five phases.[35]

- Phase 0: Exploratory study involving very limited human exposure to the drug, with no therapeutic or diagnostic goals (for example, screening studies, microdose studies)
- Phase 1: Studies are conducted with healthy volunteers, and that emphasize safety. The goal is to find out what the drug's most frequent and serious adverse events are, often, how the drug is metabolized and excreted.
- Phase 2: Studies that gather preliminary data on effectiveness (whether the drug works in people who have a disease or condition). For example, participants receiving the drug may be compared with similar participants receiving a different treatment, such as an inactive substance, called a placebo, or a different drug. In the phase, safety is evaluated continuously, and short-term adverse events are studied.

- Phase 3: Studies that gather more information about safety and effectiveness by studying different populations and different dosages and by using the drug in combination with other drugs.
- Phase 4: Studies are occurring after FDA has approved a drug for marketing. These include post-market requirement and commitment studies that are required of or agreed to by the study sponsor. These studies gather additional information about a drug's safety, efficacy, or optimal use.

Recommended sample size in a clinical trial for drug development

Current clinical trials follow a typical series of early, small-scale, from Phase 1 to late-stage, large-scale, Phase 3 studies.[36]

Phase 1: 20–100 healthy volunteers or people with the study disease or condition of interest. The purpose of Phase 1 is to test safety and dosage of a new treatment. It commonly takes several months to complete this phase.

Phase 2: Up to several hundred patients with the disease or condition of interest. The purpose of Phase 2 is to test efficacy and side effects. It commonly takes several months to 2 years to complete this phase.

Phase 3: 300–3000 volunteers who have the disease or condition of interest. The purpose of Phase 3 is to further test the efficacy and monitoring of adverse reactions in larger study participants. It commonly takes 1–4 years to complete this phase.

The above three phases are mandatory for a development of new medical products. Meanwhile, Phase 4 is under consideration and recommended by FDA.

Phase 4: Trials are carried out once the drug or device has been approved by FDA during the Post-Market Safety Monitoring. The purpose of Phase 4 is to test the safety and efficacy further using data in the real world.

Impact of clinical trials versus community trials

It is observed most clinical trials are conducted in patients with a disease or condition of interest and they are hospital-based studies. Clinical trials are necessary to test a new drug and device development that are applied in persons with the target disease or condition.

However, as we know the number of patients who receive healthcare in hospitals is much smaller than the number of persons who live in communities, they may have no clinically diagnosed disease or condition of the study interest, but they may be at subclinical stages of the disease and condition or are at high risk of the development of the disease or predisease states.[11,29,30] In the case, a community-based clinical trial may have a substantial impact on population health.

STRATEGIES FOR DATA COLLECTION

Strategies and processes for data collection and quality of control and evaluation of the data processes are the important aspects of a study.[30,31,37]

There is a common mistake that if a researcher thought that the more the data they collect, the better they have. Because if we collect the data that are unnecessary for the study's purpose, it not only increases unnecessary cost but also consumes unnecessary time. On the other hand, if we do not collect the data that we need, it will lead to an unsuccessful study as well. What data we should collect in a study are determined case by case. The following principles offer an overall strategy of data collection.

Groups of Data Collection
Outcomes
A precise definition and measurable outcome should be classified. For example, if the prognoses of patients with heart failure are the study results, the definitions of what the prognoses should be articulated, such as whether it is a 30-day readmission in patients with heart failure or 30-day in-hospital mortality.

Predictors
What are the main factors/predictors of interest should be very clear and measurable. For example, to test an education-based intervention program for the purpose of the reduction of readmission in patients with heart failure, changes in patients' adherence to medications and adherence to a healthy lifestyle may be the critical measures, because these factors predict readmission rates. Several other factors, such as the severity of disease, age, sex, and comorbidity status, may also be important predictors. It should be noted that in a hypothesis-driven scientific research, the predictors of interest needed to be focused and specified, instead of a study for a broad range of factors.

Covariates
Once the outcome(s) and predictors are classified, potential and relevant covariates (or confounders) should be classified and collected as well. They should be taken into consideration at data analysis stage as well.

SMART Approach
It is important to develop a SMART approach in data collection.[37]

SMART stands for
Specific
Measurable
Attainable/Achievable
Relevant
Time bound

Specific—What exactly are we going to collect the data for the purpose of testing our specific research questions?

Measurable—Is it quantifiable and can WE measure it?

Measurable implies the ability to count or otherwise quantify an activity or its results. It also means that the source of and mechanism for collecting measurement data are identified, and the collection of these data is feasible.

In a cohort study, a baseline measurement is required to document its change (e.g., to measure percentage increase or decrease). Following another consideration is whether the change can be measured in a meaningful and interpretable way, given the accuracy of the measurement tool and method. For example, to estimate population awareness of the signs and symptoms of heart attack, we use a sample of the state population. Because the results (such as the rate of those who know the syndrome of heart attack) come from a sample, there is a chance of error associated with the estimated value (e.g., rate). Standard instruments, such as Rose angina questionnaire, should be used.

Attainable/Achievable—Can we get it done in the proposed time frame with the resources and support we have available?

The objective and data collection approaches must be feasible with the available resources, appropriately limited in scope, and within the program's control and influence.

Relevant—Will the data being collected be appropriate for the study?

Are the relationship between the specific research questions and the overall goals of the study relevant? Evidence of relevancy can come from a literature review, best practices, or new theory and research questions to be tested.

Time bound—When will the data collection be completed?

A specified and reasonable time frame should be incorporated into the study design and specific research questions in data collection. If an intervention study (either clinical trial or community trial) is designed, it should take into consideration the environment in which the change are achievable, the scope of the change expected, and how it fits into the overall work plan.

DETERMINING THE SAMPLE SIZE
Basic Concepts
One of the most frequent questions asked by physicians when they conduct a study is "How many subjects do we have to study?" To answer this question, we need to understand the following relevant concepts:
- Effect size
- Type I error and type II error
- Probability alpha (α) and beta (β)
- Power of study

Effect size
Assume that, in a study, we know the current cure rate for patients with heart failure is 60%, and a new therapy may have a cure rate of 62%. Does the 2% difference mean the new therapy is better than the current one? Most people may consider this difference is too small to have any clinical significance, as it may occur by chance or even if it does not arise by chance. Suppose the difference between the current and new therapies is 5%, could we say the new therapy is better than the current? That would depend on how large a difference we thought is clinically meaningful. The size of the difference we want to detect is called the effect size.

Type I error and type II error
Example: A trial in which groups are receiving one of two therapies, therapy A and therapy B. Before beginning the study, we can list the four possible study results:
- The treatments are not different, and we correctly conclude that they are not different.
- The treatments are different, but we conclude that they are not different (type II error).
- The treatments are not different, but we conclude that they are different (type I error).
- The treatments are different, and we correctly conclude that they are different.
  Fig. 3.9 shows the four potential results.

Probability α and probability β

Probability α = Probability of making a type I error
= Probability of concluding the treatments are different, but in reality, they are not different
= is the $P-$value in statistical tests

In a significant test, if we set up α at $P \le .05$, this means we are willing to take the risk of a type I error at ≤5%.

Probability β = Probability of making a type II error
= Probability of concluding the treatments are not different, but in reality, they are different

Power of study
Statistical power means the probability of finding a real effect (of the size that you think is clinically relevant).

Power = $1 - \beta$
= Probability of correctly concluding that the treatments are different
= the statistical power of the study

Calculation of Sample Size
In general, to estimate a sample size, we need the following information:
- An estimate of the difference (i.e., the effect size) between the current rate and an expected rate to be detected
- Level of statistical significance (α)
- The power of study desired $(1-\beta)$
- Whether the statistical test should be one sided or two sided

Example
To calculate sample size (n) for the difference between two proportions:

$$n = \frac{(p1 * q1) + (p2 * q2)}{(p2 - p1)^2} * f(\alpha, \ power)$$

where p1 = rate in group 1, q1 = 1 − p1; p2 = rate in group 2, q2 = 1 − p2; α = significant level.

The value of (α, power) for a two-tailed test can be obtained from Table 3.4.

In a study, we know the current cure rate for patients with heart failure is 60%, and we expect a new cure rate of 75% with a new therapy. How many subjects do we have to study, with α at P-value of 0.05 and power $(1-\beta)$ of 0.80?

	Reality	
We conclude	Treatment are <u>not</u> different	Treatment <u>are</u> different
Treatment are <u>not</u> different	Correct decision	**Type II error** (β)
Treatment <u>are</u> different	**Type I error** (α)	Correct decision

FIG. 3.9 Types I and II errors.

p1 = 0.60, q1 = 0.40; p2 = 0.75, q2 = 0.25, α = 0.05, power = 0.80.

$f(α, power) = 7.9$ (from Table 3.4)

$$n = \frac{(0.60 * 0.40) + (0.75 * 0.25)}{(0.75 - 0.60)^2} * 7.9$$
$$= 150$$

The investigators would need 150 participants in each group to be 80% sure that they can detect a difference from 60% to 75% at the significant level of 0.05.

To calculate the sample size (n) for the difference between two means:

The formula to estimate sample size for a test of the difference between two means, assuming there is an equal number in each group, is:

$$n = \left[k * 2σ^2 \right] / (MD)^2$$

where $σ^2$ is the error variance, MD is the minimum difference an investigator wishes to detect, and k depends on the significance level and power desired. Selected values of k are shown in Table 3.5.

Example

To detect a difference in mean systolic blood pressure of 5 mm Hg between two groups of people, where the variance = 16^2 = 256, at a significance level of 0.05 and with a power of 0.80, then the estimated sample size:

$$N = [7.849 * 2 * (256)] / 5^2$$
$$= 161$$

That, we would need 161 participants in each group; this means that we are 80% likely to detect a difference as large or larger than 5 mm Hg.

To estimate a sample size, we may calculate using these formulas above, or use computer software to calculate it. Now, most computer software can calculate a sample size quickly as long as we have the required information.

GENERALIZABILITY OF RESULTS

Whenever we carry out a trial, the ultimate objective is to generalize the results beyond the study population itself. Two basic concepts are related to the generalizability of results: internal validity and external validity (Fig. 3.10).

Internal validity: whether the study has been done appropriately, and the findings are valid for the study sample.

External validity: whether the findings are valid for the large "reference" population.

COMMON DATA SOURCES IN HEART FAILURE STUDY

Investigators rely on many data sources for planning their research to ask specific research questions

TABLE 3.4
Values of f (α, Power)

α Significance Level	VALUE OF POWER			
	0.95	0.9	0.8	0.5
0.10	10.8	8.6	6.2	2.7
0.05	13.0	10.5	7.9	3.8
0.01	17.8	14.9	11.7	6.6

TABLE 3.5
α, Power and k Values

Significance Level	Power	k
0.05	0.99	18.372
	0.95	12.995
	0.90	10.507
	0.80	7.849
0.01	0.99	24.031
	0.95	17.814
	0.90	14.879
	0.80	11.679

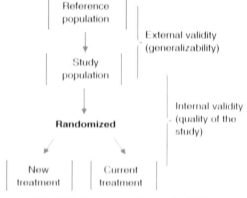

FIG. 3.10 External and internal validities.

and test specific research hypotheses. Knowing the "home" of a data source can make your research efforts substantially more efficient, representative, and meaningful. According to the nature of data collection conducted by the investigators, there are two types of data: primary data and secondary data.

Primary Data Collection

When the data collected directly by the researchers for the first time, it is called primary data. Primary data collection is necessary when a researcher cannot find the data needed. Meanwhile, the advantage of using primary data is that researchers are collecting information for the specific purposes of their study. Researchers collect the data themselves, using interviews, surveys, and direct observations. Data collection through chart reviews and/or EHR system can also be considered as primary data collection, specifically if these data are collected through the physicians themselves.

Secondary Data Collection

Secondary data collection is to obtain data from another party. There are several types of secondary data. They can include

- Population-based health surveys coordinated by the World Health Organization, such as the World Health Survey[38–40]
- Population-based health surveys conducted by national health agencies, such as the U.S. National Health and Nutrition Examination Surveys (NHANES)[41,42], and Behavior Risk Factor Surveillance System (BRFSS)[43]
- Statewide, regional, city, and community-based health surveys, such as the Southeastern Pennsylvania Household Health Surveys[44,45]

Compared with primary data, secondary data tend to be readily available and inexpensive to obtain. In addition, secondary data from state, national, and international surveys tend to have large samples, and their data collections are relatively comprehensive and representative. In the United States, several national surveys have been conducted for decades; they allow researchers to detect change over time and evaluate any impacts of change in a particular health policy, for example, the relationship between decreases in smoking rate and risk reduction of cardiovascular disease in the past decades.

An investigator may obtain a secondary dataset from the US National Institutes of Health directly, for example, from the NHLBI Biorepository and NIDDK Central Repository.[46,47]

NHLBI Biorepository

The NHLBI is one of 27 institutes and centers at the National Institutes of Health. The Institute supports basic, translational, and clinical research in heart, lung, and blood diseases. It has supported data collection from participants in epidemiology studies and clinical trials for over six decades. These data have often been sent to the NHLBI at the conclusion of the study and placed in a Data Repository. The Data Repository is managed by NHLBI staff in the DCVS Epidemiology Branch and includes individual level data on more than 580,000 participants from over 110 Institute-supported clinical trials and observational studies.[46] Fig. 3.11 depicts an overview of the access to NHLBI biospecimens and data.[48]

For example, an investigator may request data from the NHLBI repository on heart failure including the following studies:

- Heart Failure Network (HFN) CARdiorenal REScure Study in Acute Decompensated Heart Failure (CARRESS)
- Heart Failure Network (HFN) Diuretic Optimization Strategies Evaluation in Acute Heart Failure (DOSE AHF)
- Antihypertensive and Lipid-Lowering Treatment to Prevent Heart Attack Trial (ALLHAT)
- Atherosclerosis Risk in Communities (ARIC)
- Cardiovascular Health Study (CHS)
- Framingham Heart Study (FHS)

NIDDK Central Repository

The NIDDK is to conduct and support medical research and research training and to disseminate science-based information on diabetes and other endocrine and metabolic diseases; digestive diseases, nutritional disorders, and obesity; and kidney, urologic, and hematologic diseases, to improve people's health and quality of life. Several existing datasets are available on an application to conduct a secondary data analysis and or set up an ancillary study. Fig. 3.12 depicts the NIDDK Central Repository website.[47]

The following datasets, which include heart failure as an outcome and/or comorbidity, are available from the NIDDK Central Repository:

- Chronic Renal Insufficiency Cohort Study
- Look AHEAD: Action for Health in Diabetes
- Assessment, Serial Evaluation, and Subsequent Sequelae of Acute Kidney Injury (ASSESS-AKI) Study

STATISTICAL ANALYSIS STRATEGIES BY STUDY DESIGNS

Studies with different research designs and characteristics of data (in continuous or categorical) request different

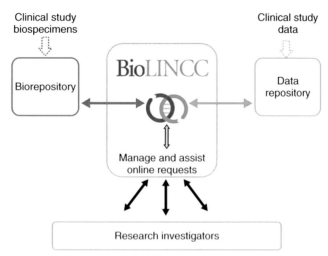

FIG. 3.11 Facilitating access to NHLBI biospecimens and data.

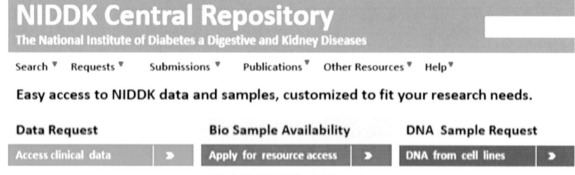

FIG. 3.12 NIDDK Central Repository.

approaches in data analysis. Table 3.6 shows the principle of data analysis strategies by research designs.

SIGNIFICANCE

Study designs are fundamental in an epidemiologic study. Several ways are used to clarify research designs. It can be descriptive epidemiologic studies and analytic epidemiology studies, or observational studies and experimental studies. No matter whatever a classification is, a study focusing on the description of the determinants and outcomes by person, place, and time is frequently applied to describe the burden of disease and risk factors. A study focusing on comparisons of the risk of disease between exposure and nonexposure groups is frequently implemented in an etiologic study, intervention study, and clinical and community trials.

Cross-sectional studies are designed to determine "what is happening?" right now. Subjects are selected, and the information is obtained at a point in time.

Case-control studies begin with the absence (i.e., controls) and presence (i.e., cases) of an outcome and then look backward in time to try to detect possible causes or risk factors that may have been suggested in descriptive studies (such as ecologic study, cross sectional study, or clinical case report). It asks, "what happened?"

Cohort studies are forward looking from a risk factor to an outcome. It asks "what will happen?"

Clinical trials, including community trials, and most of the randomized control approaches, are forward looking from a new treatment and/or intervention to outcomes. It asks, "whether it works (for the treatment and or intervention)?"

TABLE 3.6
Statistical Analysis Strategies

	ANALYSIS STRATEGIES		
Research Design	**Univariate**	**Multivariate**	**Reference Chapters**
DESCRIPTIVE STUDY			
Ecologic	Mean, frequency Simple correlation, regression Test for trend (rates)	Partial correlation Multiple regression	3 and 4 and 5
Cross sectional	Mean, frequency Simple correlation, regression Test for trend (rates)	Linear regression Logistic regression	3 and 4 and 5
ANALYTIC STUDY			
Case control	Mean, frequency Odds ratios	Logistic regression	4 3 and 4
Cohort	Mean, frequency Relative risk PAR[a] Kaplan-Meier	Cox's regression	3 and 4 3 3 5
Clinical trial	Kaplan-Meier	Cox's regression	5
Community trial	Kaplan-Meier	Cox's regression	5

[a]*PAR*, population attributable risk.

REFERENCES

1. Liu L, Nguyen C, Ariola K, et al. Action-oriented participatory intervention and outcomes in patients with heart failure: findings from the african american heart failure (pilot) study. *Circ Cardiovasc Qual Outcomes.* 2013;6(suppl 1):A310.
2. Rahman M, Pressel S, Davis BR, et al. Renal outcomes in high-risk hypertensive patients treated with an angiotensin-converting enzyme inhibitor or a calcium channel blocker vs a diuretic: a report from the Antihypertensive and Lipid-Lowering Treatment to Prevent Heart Attack Trial (ALLHAT). *Arch Intern Med.* 2005;165(8):936–946.
3. Marrero D, Pan Q, Barrett-Connor E, et al. Impact of diagnosis of diabetes on health-related quality of life among high risk individuals: the Diabetes Prevention Program outcomes study. *Qual Life Res.* 2014;23(1):75–88.
4. Khoury MJ, Gwinn M, Ioannidis JP. The emergence of translational epidemiology: from scientific discovery to population health impact. *Am J Epidemiol.* 2010;172(5):517–524.
5. Ogilvie D, Craig P, Griffin S, Macintyre S, Wareham NJ. A translational framework for public health research. *BMC Public Health.* 2009;9:116. http://dx.doi.org/10.1186/1471-2458-9-116.
6. Heymans S, Hirsch E, Anker SD, et al. Inflammation as a therapeutic target in heart failure? A scientific statement from the Translational Research Committee of the Heart Failure Association of the European Society of Cardiology. *Eur J Heart Fail.* 2009;11(2):119–129.
7. Liu L. *Racial Disparities in Pre-clinical Cardiac Abnormality and its Associations with Diabetes Mellitus and Renal Insufficiency: Translation of Research into Policy.* Paper presented at: Annual Meeting; 2007.
8. McNeil D. *Epidemiological Research Methods.* West Sussex, England: John Wiley & Sons; 1996.
9. Lash Timothy L, Fox MP, Fink Aliza K. *Applying Quantitative Bias Analysis to Epidemiologic Data.* Spring Street, New York, NY 19913, USA: Spring; 2009.
10. Schleithoff SS, Zittermann A, Tenderich G, Berthold HK, Stehle P, Koerfer R. Vitamin D supplementation improves cytokine profiles in patients with congestive heart failure: a double-blind, randomized, placebo-controlled trial. *Am J Clin Nutr.* 2006;83(4):754–759.
11. Zittermann A, Schleithoff SS, Koerfer R. Vitamin D insufficiency in congestive heart failure: why and what to do about it? *Heart Fail Rev.* 2006;11(1):25–33.
12. Zittermann A, Schleithoff SS, Tenderich G, Berthold HK, Korfer R, Stehle P. Low vitamin D status: a contributing factor in the pathogenesis of congestive heart failure? *J Am Coll Cardiol.* 2003;41(1):105–112.
13. Pilz S, Marz W, Wellnitz B, et al. Association of vitamin D deficiency with heart failure and sudden cardiac death in a large cross-sectional study of patients referred for coronary angiography. *J Clin Endocrinol Metab.* 2008;93(10):3927–3935.
14. Liu L, Chen M, Hankins SR, et al. Serum 25-hydroxyvitamin D concentration and mortality from heart failure and cardiovascular disease, and Premature mortality from all-cause in United States adults. *Am J Cardiol.* 2012;110:834–839.

15. HealthKnowledge. Causation in epidemiology: association and causation. https://www.healthknowledge.org.uk/e-learning/epidemiology/practitioners/causation-epidemiology-association-causation.

16. Szklo M, Nieto FJ. *Epidemiology beyond the Basics*. vol. 2. Sudbury, MA: Jones and Bartlett; 2007.

17. Buring CHHJE. *Epidemiology in Medicine*. Philadelphia, PA: Lippincott Williams and Wilkins; 1987.

18. Höfler M. The Bradford Hill considerations on causality: a counterfactual perspective. *Emerg Themes Epidemiol*. 2005;2(1):11.

19. National Center for Health S. *National Hospital Discharge Surveys*. vol. 2011. Hyattsville, Maryland: Public Health Service; 1980–2007.

20. Liu L. Changes in cardiovascular hospitalization and co-morbidity of heart failure in the United States: findings from the National Hospital Discharge Surveys 1980–2006. *Int J Cardiol*. 2011;149(1):39–45.

21. Mehta K, Soni R, Mehta T, Sheth K, Mansuri Z, Liu L. Influence of epidemiological risk factors in development of ventilator associated pneumonia in hospitalized patient requiring mechanical ventilation: a nationwide analysis. *CHEST J*. 2014;146(4). 218A-218A.

22. Long Y, Gracely EJ, Newschaffer CJ, Liu L. Analysis of the prevalence of cardiovascular disease and associated risk factors for European-american and african-american populations in the state of Pennsylvania 2005–2009. *Am J Cardiol*. 2013;111(1):68–72.

23. Liu L, An Y, Chen M, et al. Trends in the prevalence of hospitalization attributable to hypertensive diseases among United States adults aged 35 and older from 1980 to 2007. *Am J Cardiol*. 2013;112(5):694–699.

24. Liu L, Yang X, Long Y, et al. Changes in the prevalence of hospitalization and comorbidity in US adults with stroke: a three decade cross-sectional and birth cohort analysis. *Int J Stroke*. 2016;11(9):987–998.

25. Liu L, Ikeda K, Yamori Y. Changes in stroke mortality rates for 1950 to 1997 A great slowdown of decline trend in Japan. *Stroke*. 2001;32(8):1745–1749.

26. Lindenauer PK, Lagu T, Rothberg MB, et al. Income inequality and 30 day outcomes after acute myocardial infarction, heart failure, and pneumonia: retrospective cohort study. *BMJ*. 2013;346:f521.

27. Dunlay SM, Weston SA, Jacobsen SJ, Roger VL. Risk factors for heart failure: a population based case control study. *Am J Med*. 2009;122(11):1023–1028.

28. Stanford School of Medicine CHO Learning Modules. *Nested Case Control*. 2004. http://chiomods.stanford.edu/trailmaps/design/design/nestedCase Control/index.html.

29. Hsieh P, Hsiao F. Risk of heart failure associated with dopamine agonists: a nested case-control study. *Drugs Aging*. 2013;30(9):739–745.

30. Gordis L. *Epidemiology*. 5th ed. Toronto, Canada: Elsevier Canada; 2014.

31. Rothman K, Greenland D, Lash H. *Modern Epidemiology*. vol. 3. Philadelphia, PA: Wolters Kluwer Lippincott Williams and Wilkins; 2008.

32. National Institures of Health. Definitions of criteria and considerations for research Project grant (RPG/R01/R03/R15/R21/R34). *Critiques*. 2016. https://grants.nih.gov/grants/peer/critiques/rpg.htm.

33. Semigran MJ. *Study of Sildenafil in Advanced Heart Failure*; 2003-2006. https://clinicaltrials.gov/ct2/show/NCT00309790.

34. Lewis GD, Shah R, Shahzad K, et al. Sildenafil improves exercise capacity and quality of life in patients with systolic heart failure and secondary pulmonary hypertension. *Circulation*. 2007;116(14):1555–1562.

35. ClinicalTrials.gov. Clinical Trial Phases. https://clinicaltrials.gov/ct2/help/phase_desc.

36. U.S. Food and Drug Administration. The Drug Development Process. https://www.fda.gov/ForPatients/Approvals/Drugs/default.htm.

37. CDC Division for Heart Disease and Stroke Prevention. Evaluation Guide: Writing SMART Objectives. https://www.cdc.gov/dhdsp/programs/spha/evaluation_guides/docs/smart_objectives.pdf.

38. WHO. *World Health Organization Statistical Information System*; 2010. http://www.who.int/healthinfo/survey/en/.

39. Liu L, Ma J, Yin X, Kelepouris E, Eisen HJ. Global variability in angina pectoris and its association with body mass index and poverty. *Am J Cardiol*. 2011;107(5):655–661.

40. Liu L, Yin X, Morrissey S. Global variability in diabetes mellitus and its association with body weight and primary healthcare support in 49 low- and middle-income developing countries. *Diabet Med*. 2012;29(8):995–1002.

41. NHANES C-N. National Health and Nutrition Examination Survey Data. Hyattsville, MD: U.S. Department of Health and Human Services, Centers for Disease Control and Prevention. vol. 2010.

42. Liu L, Hankins SR, Watson RA, Weinstock PJ, Eisen HJ. Serum 25-hydroxyvitamin D concentration, heart failure mortality, and premature death from all-cause in us adults: an eight-year follow-up study. *J Card Fail*. 2010;16(8):S7.

43. Liu L, Nunez AE. Cardiometabolic syndrome and its association with education, smoking, diet, physical activity, and social support: findings from the Pennsylvania 2007 BRFSS Survey. *J Clin Hypertens (Greenwich)*. 2010;12(7):556–564.

44. Liu L, Nuñez AE. Multilevel and urban health modeling of risk factors for diabetes mellitus: a new insight into public health and preventive medicine. *Adv Prev Med*. 2014;2014.

45. Liu L, Nunez AE, Yu X, Yin X, Eisen HJ, for Urban Health Research G. Multilevel and spatial time trend analyses of the prevalence of hypertension in a large urban city in the USA. *J Urban Health*. 2013;90(6):1053–1063.

46. NHLBI BioLINCC. *Web Access to NHLBI Biospecimens and Data*; 2017. https://biolincc.nhlbi.nih.gov/home/.

47. NIDDK. *NIDDK Central Repository*; 2016. https://www.niddkrepository.org/home/.

48. NHLBI BioLINCC. *The BioLINCC Handbook*; 2016. https://biolincc.nhlbi.nih.gov/static/guidelines/handbook.pdf?link time=2017_05_08-09_58_24.847747.

CHAPTER 4

Biostatistical Basis of Inference in Heart Failure Study

BASIC STATISTICS CONCEPTS

Definition of statistics and biostatistics: Statistics is the science and art of collecting, summarizing, and analyzing data that are subject to random variation. Biostatistics is statistics applied to the life and health sciences.[1-3]

Types of Statistical Data

There are three different types of data: numerical, categorical, and ordinal data.

Numerical data

Numerical data have a meaning as a measurement, such as a person's age, weight, height, or blood pressure. Numerical data includes two subtypes of data: discrete and continuous.

- Discrete data represent items that can be counted. They take on possible values that can be listed out. For example, the number of patients with heart failure treated by a hospital each year or the number of patients who developed cardiorenal syndrome is discrete. The scale of discrete data has values equal to integers.
- Continuous data represent measurements; their possible values cannot be counted and can only be described using intervals on the real number line. For example, a person's blood pressure measures are continuous. Continuous data are always primarily numeric. The scale of continuous data has a fixed and defined interval. For example, blood pressure had a fixed and equal interval by the unit of mmHg. It is also called interval scale data.

    Data that are counted or measured using numerically defined method are called quantitative data, for example, the measures of HBA1C and ejection fraction.

Categorical data

Categorical data represent characteristics such as a person's gender, race/ethnicity, marital status, or subtypes of a disease (such as systolic HF and diastolic HF). Categorical data can take on numerical values (such as "1" indicating male and "2" indicating female), but these numbers do not have mathematical meaning. These data can be further broken into two types: dichotomous (binary) and nominal (more than two categories) variables.

Data that represent categories are also collectively called qualitative data.

Ordinal data

Ordinal data mixes numerical and categorical data. The data fall into categories, but the numbers placed on the categories have a meaning. For example, rating self-perceived health conditions on a scale from 0 (lowest) to 4 (highest) levels gives ordinal data. Ordinal data can be treated as categorical, where the groups are ordered when graphs and charts are made. However, unlike categorical data, the numbers do have mathematical meaning. For example, heart failure stages A to D represents the development of the disease toward more severity.

Changes from Continuous Data to Categorical Data

In data analysis and clinical practice, we may convert a continuous variable to a categorical variable based on a specific research and/or practice of interest. For example, blood pressure can be categorized based on the clinical cutoff points: hypertension is defined if a person has systolic blood pressure (SBP) of ≥ 140 mm Hg or diastolic blood pressure (DBP) of ≥ 90 mm Hg. When categorizing a continuous variable to a categorical variable (including dichotomized or multiple ranked variables), standard clinical references and/or recommendations by professional associations/organizations are commonly applied for setting up the cutoff points. For example, subjects with serum hemoglobin A1c (HBA1c) $\geq 5.7\%$ and HBA1c $< 6.5\%$ are classified as having prediabetes, and those with HBA1c $\geq 6.5\%$ are classified as having diabetes. In case, if a commonly acceptable cutoff point for a continuous variable is not available, one may categorize this variable based on its quantile distributions in the study population, or either by every 1, or, 5 or 10 unit interval as the cutoff points.

DESCRIPTIVE BIOSTATISTICS
Definition
Descriptive biostatistics targets about the measures of central tendency (mean, median, mode), the measures of dispersion (standard deviation [SD], the coefficient of variation, range, quartile deviation), and the measures of frequency.

Measures of Central Tendency and Variation
Central tendency
In statistics, a central tendency is a central or typical value for a probability distribution. The most common measures of central tendency are the arithmetic mean, the median, and the mode, although geometric mean is also used frequently in the medical field as well.

Arithmetic mean
Arithmetic mean ($\overline{X}$), or commonly called mean, is the arithmetic average of the observations. Example: consider the following ages for a small sample of 10 people ($n = 10$): 11, 13, 15, 17, 20, 22, 24, 25, 27, 32.

$$\overline{X} = \sum X/n = (11 + 13 + 15 + 17 + 20 + 22 + 24 + 25 + 27 + 32)/10$$
$$= 206/10$$
$$= 20.6 \text{ (the average age in years for the 10 people)}$$

Median
Median is the middle observation that is the point at which half the observations are smaller, and half are larger. To determine the median, order the data from low to high, we use the example (still use the 10 numbers above): 11, 13, 15, 17, 20, 22, 24, 25, 27, 32.

Median = $(20 + 22)/2 = 21$ (the median age for the 10 people).

Mode
The mode is the value that occurs most frequently. It is commonly used for a large number of observations when the researcher wants to designate the value that occurs most often.

Example 1 (still using the previous data set): 11, 13, 15, 17, 20, 22, 24, 25, 27, 32.

Can we get the model from the data above? NO, because no value appears more than once in this dataset, it has no mode.

Example 2: suppose data values are 2, 6, 7, 8, 8, 6, 5, 1, 3, and 8.

Here the mode is 8 because this value appears three times; it is the most frequent one.

Geometric mean
The geometric mean is the nth root of the product of n numbers. It is commonly used in data measured on a logarithmic scale, such as the dilution of smallpox vaccine.

For example, for a set of numbers, X1, X2, X3, ... Xn, the geometric mean is calculated as below.

$$\text{Geometric mean} = \sqrt[n]{X1 * X2 * X3 * \cdots Xn}$$

Measures of spread
Although means (i.e., $\overline{X}$ and median) provide useful information of the central tendency of a dataset, we could have a better idea of the distribution of data if we know something about the spread. The most common measures of spread include SD, coefficient of variation, percentiles, and interquartile range. These measures are based on deviations from the mean.

Standard deviation
SD: It represents the average deviation of each observation from the mean.

$$SD = \sqrt{\frac{SS}{(n-1)}} = \sqrt{S^2}$$

$$SS \text{ (the sum of squares)} = \sum (x - \overline{X})^2$$

S^2: Variance

Example (still use the previous data set): $n = 10$, and mean = 20.6.
11, 13, 15, 17, 20, 22, 24, 25, 27, 32.

$$\text{Then, } SS = (11 - 20.6)^2 + (13 - 20.6)^2 + (15 - 20.6)^2 + \cdots + (32 - 20.6)^2$$
$$= 398.3$$

$$SD = \sqrt{398.3/(10 - 1)}$$
$$= 6.65 \text{ (years)}$$

Conclusion: $n = 10$, $\overline{X} = 20.6$ (years), and SD = 6.65 (years)

Coefficient of variation
The coefficient of variation (CV) is defined as the SD divided by the mean times 100%. It is a useful measure of *relative spread* in data (when these data have different units of measurements). By using this formula below, we eliminate the different units of measures and can compare the spread of various types of measures.

$$CV = \frac{SD}{\overline{X}} * 100$$

Example. In a study sample, we get mean SBP (mm Hg), $\overline{X} = 137.86$, and SD = 21.22.
Mean HBA1c (%), $\overline{X} = 5.88$, and SD = 1.26

If we want to compare the variability of individuals on the two different measures, we need to compare their relative spread (i.e., CV) because each measure has its different measurement scales.

$$CV\ (SBP) = \frac{21.22}{137.86} * 100 = 15.39\%$$

$$CV\ (HBA1c) = \frac{1.26}{5.88} * 100 = 21.42\%$$

Interpretation, the relative variation HBA1c for people in the sample, is considerately greater than the variation in SBP.

Percentiles

A percentile is the percentage of a distribution that is equal to or below a particular number. For example, the 50th percentile has the same value as the median.

Interquartile range

A measure of variation that makes use of percentiles, defined as the difference between the 25th and 75th percentiles, is also called the first and third quartiles, respectively. For example, among the 10 observations: 11, 13, 15, 17, 20, 22, 24, 25, 27, 32, the 25th percentile = 15 and the 75th percentile = 25.

Another measure of spread: range

The range is the difference between the largest and the smallest observation.

Example, among the 10 observations: 11, 13, 15, 17, 20, 22, 24, 25, 27, 32.

The range = 32 − 11 = 21.

SAS Computing

Introduction to easy-to-use SAS

What SAS stands for?. SAS stands for "Statistical Analysis System," was developed in the early 1970s at North Carolina State University. It was originally intended for management and analysis of agricultural field experiments, but now it is the most widely used statistical software across the multiple disciplinary, including medicine and public health.[4,5]

Since the 1970s, SAS has developed more than 200 components, sometimes called products, to meet the needs of a growing requirement across all the sciences. The following is an overall list of the most used SAS products.[4]

- Base SAS—Basic procedures and data management
- SAS/STAT—Statistical analysis
- SAS/GRAPH—Graphics and presentation
- SAS/OR—Operations Research

- SAS/ETS—Econometrics and Time Series Analysis
- SAS/IML—Interactive matrix language
- SAS/AF—Applications facility
- SAS/QC—Quality control
- SAS/INSIGHT—Data mining
- SAS/PH—Clinical trial analysis
- Enterprise Miner—data mining
- Enterprise Guide—GUI based code editor & project manager
- SAS EBI—Suite of Business Intelligence Applications
- SAS Grid Manager—Manager of SAS grid computing environment

In the section, we review the basic of SAS statement and steps, and then go straight forward to reading and conduct statistics analysis using sample datasets. Readers with minimum experience in using SAS, or just a beginner, should be able to go through the examples (the SAS sample datasets and programs are available on request. Please write to me at LL85@Drexel.edu, I will get back to you immediately.)

SAS environment

Fig. 4.1A shows two important windows, the Log window and Program window (for writing Data statement and Proc statement). SAS Log window is very useful for you to monitoring and checking any programs that you have submitted are going through or have errors for action. In the Program window, it allows you to write Data statement and Procedure (Proc) statement.

Fig. 4.1B show the basic of SAS Output and Program windows. For example, in the Program window, "Libname HFBK 'C:\Book_2017\HF_Book\SASDATA';" means we create a temporal library, named "HFBK," and tell the corresponding folder where the SAS dataset is.

The data statement (DATA HFBK1; SET HFBK. HFBKBG1; RUN;") means to read SAS dataset (named HFBKBG1 from the Library HFBK). Then having the read data (HFBKBG1) named as HFBKBG1.

The Proc statement (PROC FREQ DATA=HFBKBG1; TABLES SEX; RUN;) tells SAS to run and have a Frequency table. The results show in the Output window. It indicates that in the dataset (HFBKBG1), the total sample size is 3000. Of them, 47.07% (n=1412) are males (sex=1) and 52.93% (n=1588) are females (sex=2).

SAS statement in general

SAS statements can be in upper or lower case and may begin on any column. SAS statements may also extend across lines, and more than one SAS statement may appear on a single line. SAS statements always end with a semicolon (;)

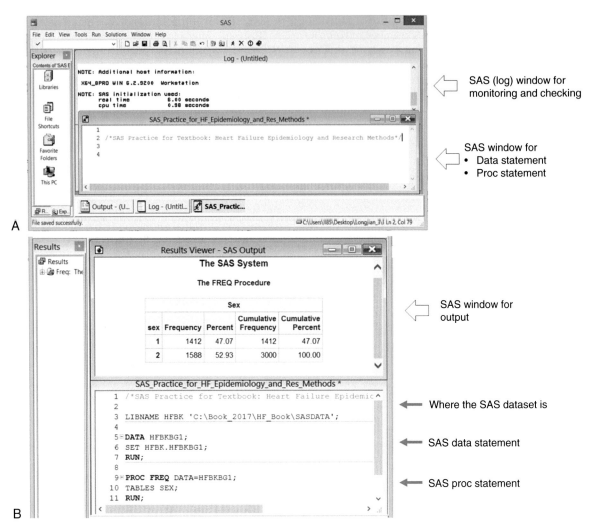

FIG. 4.1 SAS computing.

SAS Statement by Steps

- DATA step
- PROC step

There are two general steps in SAS.

The first is the **DATA** step in which data are read in, manipulated, edited, etc. The second is the **PROC** or procedure step in which some statistical procedure (e.g., MEANS, ANOVA) is performed on the data. Any number of DATA and PROC steps can occur in a single program. For example, one can create and read a dataset in the **DATA step**, then perform a mean procedure (PROC MEANS) in the **PROC step** that calculates and outputs mean, SD, minimum and maximum or specify mean, SD, percentiles, or the maximum number of decimals in the **PROC** step.

For example: In a Data step, we create an SAS dataset named as HFBK1.

Start with SAS

Estimate means. SAS practice 1

To estimate the mean of "11, 13, 15, 17, 20, 22, 24, 25, 27, 32" using SAS:

SAS Data step: Create an SAS dataset.

```
Data HFBKS101A;        ← Create a new dataset, named as 'HFBKS101A'.
Input ID AGE ;         ← Assign variable name (i.e., ID and age).
Datalines;             ← Under the datalines, '1,2,3....' represents the ID number
1  11                     of each individual. '11,13,15...' indicates the corresponding
2 13                      values of age. For example, an individual with ID number 1,
3 15                      his/her age is 11.
4 17
5 20
6 22
7 25
8 27
9 24
10 32
;
```

SAS Proc step

In the PROC MEANS step below, "MAXDEC=2" asks output values with two decimals.

PROC MEANS MAXDEC=2 DATA =HFBKS101A;
VAR AGE;
RUN;

OUTPUT 1

Analysis Variable: AGE

N	Mean	SD	Minimum	Maximum
10	20.60	6.65	11.00	32.00

Of the 10 observations, the mean is 20.6, the SD is 6.65, and the minimum and maximum values are 11 and 32.

Using the same dataset, we can select more statistics in the proc mean, such as SD, median, model, 25th and 75th percentiles, range, min and max values.

From OUTPUT 1, one may request specified statistics, such as median, percentiles 25, 75, and the number of decimals. See SAS practice 2.

SAS practice 2

PROC MEANS N MEAN STD MEDIAN P25 P75 RANGE MIN MAX MAXDEC=2 DATA =HFBKS101A;
VAR AGE;
RUN;

OUTPUT 2

Analysis Variable: AGE

N	Mean	Std Dev	Median	25th Percentile	75th Percentile	Range	Minimum	Maximum
10	20.60	6.65	21.00	15.00	25.00	21.00	11.00	32.00

Of the 10 observations, the median is 21.00, the 25th and 75th percentiles are 15 and 25, and the range is 21. However, there is no output for mode, because there is no "mode" in the original dataset (HFBKS101A).

SAS practice 3

To calculate mean, median, and mode:

To get a mode value, we need to work with a new dataset because practice 2 dataset (HFBKS101A) has no mode. An example dataset is created and named as HFBKS1B using SAS data step.

SAS Data step: Create an SAS dataset

```
Data HFBKS1B;
Input ID VALUE;
Datalines;
1  2
2  6
3  7
4  8
5  8
6  6
7  5
8  1
9  3
10 8
;
```

SAS Proc step

```
PROC MEANS N MEAN MEDIAN MODE MIN MAX MAXDEC =0 DATA =HFBKS101B;
VAR VALUE;
RUN;
```

Output

Analysis Variable: Value

N	Mean	Median	Mode	Minimum	Maximum
10	5	6	8	1	8

Of the 10 observations, the mean is 5, the median is 6, the mode is 8, and the minimum and maximum values are 1 and 8.

SAS practice 4.

To calculate mean, SD, and CV using dataset HFBKS101A:

```
PROC MEANS N MEAN STD CV MAXDEC=2 MIN MAX DATA =HFBKS101A;
VAR AGE;
RUN;
```

OUTPUT 4

Analysis Variable: AGE

N	Mean	Std Dev	Coeff of Variation	Minimum	Maximum
10	20.60	6.65	32.30	11.00	32.00

SAS computing in data with a large sample size

It should be noted that in most studies we work with large-scale datasets. We use an example sampling dataset from a large cross-sectional study, named as "HFBKBG1." This dataset is applied here for the demonstrations of SAS computing only; it is not necessary to interpret the results as any representative findings. In the sample dataset, it had 3000 participants (i.e., n = 3000).

Table 4.1 shows the first 10 observations of the dataset. The names and their codes are shown below.

STUDYID: ID number of each observation.
SEX: 1 = male, 2 = female
AGE: Age in years.
REGIONS: 1 = rural, 2 = urban
SMK: Smoking status, 0 = never smoked,
            1 = former smoked, 2 = current smokers
BMI: Body mass index, kg/m^2
SBP: Systolic blood pressure, mmHg
DBP: Diastolic blood pressure, mmHg
HF: Heart failure, 0 = No, 1 = Yes
DM: Diabetes, 0 = No, 1 = Yes
DEATH: All-cause mortality, 0 = alive, 1 = died
P_Year: Year of follow-up (person-year)

TABLE 4.1
The First 10 Observations in Dataset HFBKBG1

STUDYID	SEX	AGE	REGION2	SMK	BMI	SBP	DBP	HF	DM	DEATH	P_year
1	1	48	1	0	25	120	70	0	1	1	17.2
2	2	56	1	1	37	128	73	0	0	0	21.2
3	1	63	1	2	31.1	137	68	0	0	1	12
4	1	60	2	2	20.4	135	85	0	0	0	21.2
5	1	58	1	2	19.7	105	64	0	0	1	20.2
6	1	90	2	0	24.2	158	74	0	0	1	3.3
7	1	72	2	0	25.5	169	84	0	0	1	13.7
8	2	45	1	2	24.2	103	67	0	0	0	22.8
9	1	84	2	1	25.5	151	46	0	0	1	2.8
10	1	69	2	1	24	130	65	0	0	1	2.5

PRACTICE
Research question:
What are the mean, SD, CV, min, and max values for age, BMI, SBP, and HBA1c?
  SAS Data step: Read SAS data in

DATA HFBKBG2;
SET HFBKBG1;
RUN;
SAS Proc step

```
PROC MEANS N MEAN STD CV MIN MAX NMISS MAXDEC=2 DATA = HFBKBG2;
VAR AGE BMI SBP HBA1C;
RUN;
```

Output 5

The MEANS Procedure

Variable	N	Mean	Std Dev	Coeff of Variation	Minimum	Maximum	N Miss
age	3000	66.03	12.25	18.55	45.00	90.00	0
bmi	2643	27.36	5.57	20.35	12.80	67.30	357
sbp	2913	137.86	21.22	15.39	81.00	244.00	87
HbA1c	2553	5.88	1.26	21.42	3.70	16.20	447

The results indicate that, of the 3000 observations, the mean age (SD) was 66.03 (12.25). There were no missing values for age. The mean (SD) body mass index (BMI) was 27.36 (5.57). There were 357 missing values for BMI (3000–2643). Similar interpretations for SBP and HBA1c can be made.

Measures of Diseases Occurrence and Existence
Number of cases, crude and age-specific rates
Three factors should be considered when measuring how a disease occurs in a group of populations: (1) the number of people who are affected by the disease (or those who are diagnosed to have the disease); (2) the number of the population from which the cases of disease arise; and (3) the length of time that the population is followed.

Therefore, there are four common measures of disease occurrence: (1) counts, (2) proportion, (3) ratio, and (4) rate.

Count
The count is the number of cases of an event (e.g., those who have the disease of study interest).

Proportion
The number of cases (numerator) is a "proportion" of the number of total observations (denominator). It indicates the magnitude of a part related to the total sample (observations).

Example. A/(A + B)
Proportions, also known as fractions, are often expressed as percentages. It ranges from 0% to 100%.

For example, the proportion of patients with stage A heart failure in a sample of heart failure with stages A to D is the number of heart failure patients with stage A divided by the total number of patients with heart failure from all stages (A, B, C, and D).

Ratio
Basically, a ratio is a comparison of the count of two elements. The numerator and denominator need not be related.

Example. Male/female ratio.

Rate
It commonly indicates the measures of disease incidence, prevalence, morbidity, and mortality.

Measures of disease frequency characterize the number of persons in a population who become ill (incidence, i.e., new cases) or are ill at a given time (prevalence, i.e., currently existed cases at the study point in time), or mortality in a given period.

A rate (incidence, prevalence, and mortality) can be estimated from a sample population (crude rates). It is the actual rate of the study population. Crude rates are helpful in determining the disease burden and specific needs for services in a given population, compared with another population, regardless of size.

Incidence
Number of NEW cases of a disease occurring in the population during a specified period. There are two types of incidence measures
- Cumulative incidence rate
- Incidence density

Cumulative incidence rate: the number of new cases of disease occurring over a specified period in a population at risk at the beginning of the interval.

Incidence density (also called incidence rate): the number of new cases of disease occurring over a specified period in a population at risk throughout the interval, in which the denominator consists of the sum of the different times that an individual was at risk. The denominator is often expressed in person-time (such as person-month and person-year).

Incidence density incorporates time directly into the denominator. A person-time rate is calculated from a long-term cohort follow-up study, wherein enrollees are followed over time, and the occurrence of new cases of disease is documented. Therefore, the incidence rate is also called as person-time rate.

Prevalence rate

Prevalence measures the frequency of existing disease (i.e., including new and old disease) at a specified point in time (point prevalence) or over a given period (period prevalence).

$$\text{Prevalence rate } (\%) = \frac{\begin{array}{c}\text{No. of cases of disease}\\\text{present in the population}\\\text{at a specified time}\end{array}}{\begin{array}{c}\text{No. of persons in the}\\\text{population at that}\\\text{specific time}\end{array}} * 100$$

Mortality rate

Similar to the prevalence rate, the mortality rate is the number of deaths divided by the number of persons in the population at a specific point in time.

Mortality rates are the measures of disease mortality frequency characterize the number of persons in a population who die from a disease (disease-specific mortality) or died from any causes (all-cause mortality) at a given time.

Example. In a hospital, the annual heart failure specific mortality in 2016 = total number of death from heart failure in 2016 divided by the total of patients who received healthcare in the hospital in 2016.

All-cause mortality in 2016 is the total number of death from all causes divided by the number of patients who received healthcare in the hospital in 2016.

Case fatality rate

Case fatality rate (CFR) is the proportion of deaths within a defined population of interest. Case fatality rate measures the severity of the disease that causes death. For example, among a total of 200

patients with disease A, 20 of them died from the same disease within 30 days; the 30-day case fatality rate = 20/200 * 100 = 10%.

Similar to incidence rate, mortality rate and case fatality rate can be estimated by the number of deaths in a certain person-time. Again, a person-time rate is calculated from a long-term cohort follow-up study, wherein enrollees are followed over time and the occurrence of the cases of death) is documented.

Definition of person-time

Person-time is defined as a measure to combine the number of persons and their time contribution in a study. This measure is most often used as the denominator in incidence and mortality rates. It is the sum of individual units of time that the persons in the study population have been exposed or at risk of the conditions of interest, for example, person-year: It represents the year of an individual who has been exposed or at risk of the condition of interest.

Specific rate and total (crude) rate

Rates can be calculated for the entire sample of participants in a study (e.g., total or crude incidence, prevalence and mortality rates) or within a specific subpopulation (e.g., age-specific, sex-specific, race/ethnicity-specific, occupational-specific rates).

Example. Table 4.2 shows a hypothetical sample to demonstrate the calculations of total and age-specific prevalence of heart failure in hypothesized urban and rural areas.

In Table 4.2, the age-specific prevalence rate (per 100) in those aged 45–54 years equals the total number of cases (e.g., heart failure, n = 45) divided by the total number of those aged 45–54 who are at risk of heart failure (n = 1500) = 45/1500 * 100 = 3%.

$$\text{Total prevalence rate } (\%) = 189/3000 * 100 = 6.3\%$$

The total rate is also called crude rate because it is an overall rate among the total observations of the study.

However, comparing the rate between two (or more than two) samples, which are from two (or more) geographically different places, using total (crude) rates may cause errors because of their different age distributions. In the following sections, we introduce age-standard rates.

Age-Standardized (Adjusted) Rates

When comparing two or more than two rates, such as incidence, prevalence, or mortality rates between two (or more) populations, such as residents living in rural

TABLE 4.2
A Hypothetical Example of Age-specific Prevalence of Heart Failure (HF) in Urban and Rural Areas

| | PREVALENCE OF HEART FAILURE BY AGE IN RURAL AND URBAN | | | | | |
| | URBAN | | | RURAL | | |
Age (years)	Population (a)	HF (b)	Rate (c) = (b)/(a)	Population (d)	HF (e)	Rate (f) = (e)/(d)
45–54	1500	45	0.03	400	10	0.025
55–64	1000	89	0.089	600	42	0.07
≥65	500	55	0.11	2000	201	0.101
Total	3000	189	0.063	3000	253	0.084

Example:
Age-specific rate in years 45–54 in urban = 45/1500 * 100 = 3%
Total rate in urban = 189/3000 * 100 = 6.3%
Total rate in rural = 253/3000 * 100 = 8.4%

and urban areas, the age composition of the populations must be taken into account. Most diseases, no matter their incidence, prevalence, and/or mortality, are strongly correlated with age. Older people have higher incidence, prevalence, and mortality rates for most chronic diseases, such as coronary heart disease, heart failure, and cancer. If a population is heavily weighted by older people, its total incidence, prevalence, and/or mortality rates would be higher than that in a younger population, and a comparison between the two populations might just reflect the difference in age distribution rather than an intrinsic difference in these compared rates. There are two ways to deal with this problem when a rate is compared between two different populations.
• Compare age-specific rates
• Compare age-standardized (i.e., age-adjusted) rates
    Two age-standardization methods are used, characterized by whether the standard used is a population distribution (direct method) or a set of specific rates (indirect method).

Compare age-specific rates
For example, Table 4.3 is an extended table from Table 4.2. It shows a hypothetical example of the prevalence of heart failure in subjects aged 45 and older in urban and rural areas. The prevalence of heart failure was lower in the urban residents than that in the rural residents (6.3% vs. 8.4%) (in the left side of the table). However, when we look at age-specific rates (by age groups 45–54, 55–64, and ≥65), they were higher in urban residents (3.0%,

8.9%, and 11.0%) than that in rural residents (2.5%, 7.0%, and 10.1%). Therefore, a correct comparison should compare the age-specific rates, instead of the total rates (i.e., crude rates), or apply age-standardization methods to compare age-standardized (i.e., age-adjusted) rates.

Direct standardization method
Age-standardization rates. From the hypothetical example, Table 4.3, we can see that the difference between crude and age-specific rates is because the age structure of the population is different in the two populations (urban and rural). The prevalence is the highest in the oldest age groups (11.0% in urban and 10.1% in rural). However, the sample size of the oldest age group was much smaller in the urban study population (n = 500, 17% of the total study sample) than that in the rural (n = 2000, 67% of the total sample), Fig. 4.2. The purpose of the direct age standardization is to make the age composition of the populations the same between the two groups (urban and rural) and then to make a comparison.

Steps for direct standardization method

Example
Step 1: to select a standard population. The standard population can be selected from US census (such as 2000 or 2010 data), or from one of the study population (such as the samples in urban or rural), or from a combined total sample of the total sample (such as the total sample of urban and rural populations). The standard population selected should be by age specific groups that match what you are interested in your

study. In the example, we used the combined total sample by three age groups as the standard population. As Table 4.3 (right side) shows, the numbers of the standard population by three age groups (45–54, 55–64, and ≥65 years older) are 1900, 1600, and 2500, respectively.

Step 2: to calculate the expected number of disease
Example. The expected number of disease in those aged 45–54 in urban residents
= the number of age-specific population × the corresponding age-specific rate
= 1900 × 0.03
= 57

The expected number of disease in those aged 45–54 in rural residents
= the number of age-specific population × the corresponding age-specific rate
= 1900 × 0.025
= 48

Similar to the above calculation, we get the expected number of individuals they would have the disease according to their actual age-specific rates and the selected standard population.

TABLE 4.3
A Hypothetical Example of Age-Specific Prevalence of Heart Failure (HF) in Urban and Rural Areas, and Age-Adjusted Rates of HF (Calculated Using Direct Method)

Age (years)	PREVALENCE OF HEART FAILURE BY AGE IN RURAL AND URBAN						EXPECTED NO. OF DISEASE A		
	URBAN			RURAL			Standard	Urban	Rural
	Population (a)	HF (b)	Rate (c)=(b)/(a)	Population (d)	HF (e)	Rate (f)=(e)/(d)	Population (g)	HF h=(g)*(c)	HF (i)=(g)*(f)
45–54	1500	45	0.03	400	10	0.025	1900	57	48
55–64	1000	89	0.089	600	42	0.07	1600	142	112
≥65	500	55	0.11	2000	201	0.101	2500	275	251
Total	3000	189	**0.063**	3000	253	**0.084**	6000		
							Total expected	474	411

Age-adjusted rate:
In urban, rate=474/6000*100=7.90%
In rural, rate=411/6000*100=6.85%

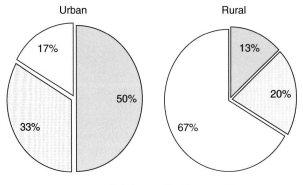

FIG. 4.2 Percentage of patients by age groups in urban and rural areas (a hypothetical dataset).

Step 3: To calculate the age-standardized rate
Example.

Age-standardized rate = the total expected number of
disease/the total standard population

Age-standardized rate in urban residents = 474/6000 * 100
= 7.90%

Age-standardized rate in rural residents = 411/6000 * 100
= 6.85%

The results indicate that age-standardized prevalence of heart failure was higher in urban residents than that in rural (7.90% vs. 6.85%). The results are consistent with that if we compare their age-specific rates (i.e., urban residents had higher age-specific heart failure rates than rural residents).

It should be noted that, when interpreting an age-standardized rate, the following issues should be kept in mind.

- Age-standardized rates are used to compare "total rates" (i.e., incidence, prevalence, or mortality rates).
- Because of the method of computation, the age-standardized rates are used for the purpose of comparison between two (or more) populations. However, they are not the "real" rates of the study populations. It represents that the observed age-specific rates were present in a population whose age distribution is that of the standard population.
- Changes in the selection of the standard population will change the values of the age-standardized rates, but the trend (i.e., higher or lower) is the same. It is important to note that, to compare two (or more) age-standardized rates, the same standard population must have been used.
- In most official reports of the US age-standardized (i.e., age-adjusted) rates (incidence, prevalence, or mortality rates) are commonly calculated according to the year 2000 population as the standard population. It offers the opportunity to compare rates directly across the states and/or counties.

Indirect standardization method

In the direct standardization method, the observed age-specific rates and a standard population are used. For indirect standardization, the observed population and a standard set of age-specific rates are used. Indirect standardization method is not used as frequency as direct standardization, but it is more often used to present a standard mortality rate (SMR) when the number of death by age-specific age groups is not available in the study population of interest. The indirect standardized rate and SMR are defined as the following.

$$SMR = \frac{\text{Number of observed deaths}}{\text{Number of expected death}} \times 100$$

Table 4.4 shows a hypothetical example of heart failure mortality in a population who were exposed to a particular occupation. The research question is whether this group of individuals had a different mortality rate than that in general population. In the case,

---

TABLE 4.4
A Hypothetical Example of Mortality Rate (per 1000) in Heart Failure (HF) Patients Exposure to a Specific Occupation (i.e., Occupation a) After an Average 12-years of follow-up

Age (years)	Estimated Population for HF Patients With Occupation A (a)	Death Rate (per 1000) in HF Patients in General Population (b)	Expected Death in HF Patients in Occupation A if They Had the Same Risk as HF Patients in General Population (c) = (a) × (b)	Observed Number of Deaths in HF Patients With Occupation A (d)
45–54	2000	53.2	106	NA
55–64	2400	67.8	163	NA
>65	2000	72.1	144	NA
Total	6400		413	550
			SMR = 550/413 * 100 = 133.17	

NA, not available; *SMR*, standard mortality rate.
The results indicate that this group of heart failure patients with occupation A had a risk of mortality 33% greater than patients with heart failure in general population.

if we had no information on the number of death by age group, but had the total number of death, and the number of the population who are at risk by the age group (i.e., the number of population by age for those with the particular occupation). We can calculate the SMR to compare the observed total number of death with the total number of mortality that we expected. The indirect age-standardization method has three steps.

Step 1: To select a standardized rate. Table 4.4 shows the death rate (per 1000) among the general population in patients with heart failure (a hypothetical example) by age groups (53.2, 67.8, and 72.1 per 1000). In the example, we select it as the standardized rate to calculate the SMR.

Step 2: To calculate the expected number of death.

The expected number of death in ages $45-54 = 2000 \times 0.0532$
$$= 106$$

The expected number of death in ages $55-64 = 2400 \times 0.0678$
$$= 163$$

The expected number of death in ages $\geq 65 = 2000 \times 0.0721$
$$= 144$$

Step 3: To calculate SMR.

SMR = (Total observed number of death/
total expected number of death) $\times 100$
$= (555/413) \times 100$
$= 133.17$

The result indicates that patients with heart failure who have an exposure to a particular occupation had a risk of mortality 33% greater than patients with heart failure in general population.

Like the direct age-standardization method, when interpreting SMR, the following should be kept in mind.
- SMR is often used when numbers of deaths for each age-specific group are not available.
- It is commonly used to study mortality in an occupationally exposed population.
- Select age- and disease-specific death rates for the general population are used as "standard."
- Numbers of age-specific population in a "target" (i.e., occupation) population are used.
- Calculate the number of total expected deaths for an occupation according to the death rate of general population.
- When comparing two populations, the SMR for each can be calculated using the same "standard" mortality rates and the SMR can be compared.

SAS Computing

In the practice, we use SAS dataset: HFBKBG1.

To calculate sex-specific rates using SAS Proc Freq

Dataset: HFBKG1

To calculate the prevalence of heart failure in males and females using SAS Proc statement:

Proc Freq.

```
PROC FREQ DATA = HFBKBG1;
TABLES SEX*HF /NOCOL;
RUN;
```

In the SAS Proc above, "NOCOL" means without the output of column percentages, because we are interested in estimating the prevalence of heart failure by sex.

The FREQ Procedure				
Frequency Percent Row Pct	Table of sex by HF			
		HF		
	sex(Sex)	NO	YES	Total
	M	1301 43.37 92.14	111 3.70 7.86	1412 47.07
	F	1486 49.53 93.58	102 3.40 6.42	1588 52.93
	Total	2787 92.90	213 7.10	3000 100.00

Interpret: The prevalence of heart failure was 7.86% in males and 6.42% in females.

Calculate Person-Year Rates

In the above, the prevalence and mortality rates we calculated are based on the baseline of HFBKBG1. In the baseline analysis, we analyze the data cross sectionally.

In a prospective study, however, like the example dataset, HFBKBG1, we need to calculate person-time (days, months, or years) when we estimate their mortality rates (from baseline to the end of follow-up).

To demonstrate how to calculate a person-time rate, suppose, an investigator conducted a prospective study and followed five patients with heart failure from baseline for up to 12 months. The results (outcomes of the five patients) are graphically displayed in Fig. 4.3.

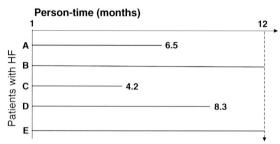

Person-time (months)

FIG. 4.3 A hypothetical cohort for person-time (months) calculation. **(A–E)** represent five patients with heart failure at baseline. They were followed for 12 months. Three of them **(A, C and D)** died within the follow up.

The graph shows how many months were followed for each patient as a case and their outcome (alive or dead). From this graph, we can calculate the person-time. The person-time is the sum of total time contributed by all patients in the follow-up study. The unit for person-time in the example is person-month.

Month contributed by each patient:

Patients A: 6.5 months
Patients B: 12 months
Patients C: 4.2 months
Patients E: 8.3 months
Patients D: 12 months

$$\text{Total person-months in the example}$$
$$= 6.5 + 12 + 4.2 + 8.3 + 12$$
$$= 43$$

The total number of death during the 12-month follow-up was 3 (A, C, and D). Therefore,

$$\text{The mortality rate} = 3/43 \text{ person-months}$$
$$= 0.06977$$
$$= 6.98 \text{ person 100 person months}$$

SAS Computing—To estimate person-time.

In DATA STEP—To create a new dataset for the hypothetical example (Fig. 4.3) of five cases.

Dataset name: HFBKPM
ID: participant's ID
TIME: Follow up time (months)
Status: 1 – died, 0 – alive

```
DATA HFBKPM;
INPUT ID TIME STATUS ;
DATAL
1 6.5 1
2 12 0
3 4.2 1
4 8.3 1
5 12 0
;
```

SAS PROC

```
PROC MEANS N MEAN STD SUM MAXDEC=2 DATA = HFBKPM;
VAR TIME;
TITLE 'PERSON-MONTHS';
RUN;
```

Output 2

	Analysis Variable: TIME		
N	Mean	Std Dev	Sum
5	8.60	3.43	43.00

The sum represents the total person-months (43).

Risk Assessments

In Measures of Diseases Occurrence and Existence section, we discussed measures of disease frequencies. For example, we apply incidence rate to describe the risk of disease (i.e., the occurrence of disease) and apply prevalence rate to describe the burden of disease (i.e., the present of disease). In this section, we discuss risk factors of disease. To determine the magnitude of an association between exposures (risk factors) and outcomes (disease) compared with those without or with limited exposure to the study of a risk factor, we commonly measure two group risk indicators: (1) absolute risk, risk difference, relative risk, and odds ratio; (2) attributable risks and population attributable risk.

Absolute risk, risk difference, and relative risk
Absolute risk. Absolute risk is the incidence of a disease in a population. Incidence rates and risk statements can also be calculated for subgroups of the population defined by some characteristics.

However, incidence does not indicate whether the exposure is associated with an increased risk of the disease because it does not take into consideration the risk of disease in nonexposed individuals. A typical research question is whether two groups (exposed vs. nonexposed) have the same probability of contracting a disease. To summarize the information (i.e., *to estimate the risk association*), we can calculate:

- Risk Difference
- Relative risk (RR)

Risk difference = (Disease risk in exposed group) −
                 (Disease risk in non-exposed group)

Relative risk = (Disease risk in exposed group) /
               (Disease risk in non-exposed group)

Table 4.5 is a hypothetical example of the incidence of heart failure in subjects with or without metabolic

TABLE 4.5
A Hypothetical Example of Incidence Rate of Heart Failure (HF) in Subjects With or Without Metabolic Syndrome (MetS)

| Exposure Status | No. of Study Participants | DISEASE STATUS | | Incidence Rate (per 1000) |
		Incident HF	Non-HF	
Individuals with MetS	2000	35	1945	17.5
Individuals without MetS	6000	65	5935	10.83
Total	8000	100	7900	12.5

MetS is defined when a subject has three or more components of five risk factors of cardiometabolic disorders: elevated waist circumference (WC > 102 cm in males and WC > 88 cm in females), elevated triglycerides (TG ≥ 150 mg/dL), decreased high-density lipoprotein cholesterol (HDL < 40 mg/dL in males and HDL < 50 mg/dL in females), elevated blood pressure (SBP ≥ 130 mm Hg or DBP ≥ 85 mm Hg), and elevated fasting glucose (≥110 mg/dL).

syndrome. Metabolic syndrome (MetS) has been identified as an independent risk for heart failure and the other main forms of cardiovascular diseases (i.e., coronary heart disease and stroke).[6]

According to the hypothetical example, we can calculate:

The absolute risk of incident heart failure in individuals with MetS was 17.5 per 1000 population (35/2000) and 10.83 per 1000 population (65/6000) in individuals without MetS.

$$\text{Risk difference} = \text{Absolute risk reduction}$$
$$= 17.5 - 10.83 = 6.67$$

$$\text{Relative risk} = 17.5/10.83 = 1.62$$

Interpretation: the risk of heart failure is 1.62 times greater among individual with MetS than those without MetS. In other words, individuals with MetS have 62% increased the risk of heart failure.

Odds ratios

It should be noted that regarding study design, data from Table 4.5 can be treated from a study that applied a prospective study design. However, when data from studies with a cross-sectional or case-control study design, the incidence is not available. Therefore, odds ratios are used to estimate RRs. In Chapter 3, we discussed 2 × 2 table and prevalence of heart failure in subjects with or without diabetes from a cross-sectional study of total 3000 participants (see Chapter 3, Tables 3.1 and 3.2).

In a cross-sectional and case-control study (see Chapter 3 Table 3.2), we calculate odds ratios between the exposure and nonexposure groups.

$$\text{Odds ratios} = a/b \div c/d$$
$$= a \times d/b \times c$$

Example. To examine the odds ratios of heart failure in patients with diabetes versus those without diabetes, as shown Chapter 3, Table 3.1:

$$\text{Odds ratios} = 70 \times 2441/143 \times 346$$
$$= 3.45$$

The results suggest that patients with diabetes had 3.45 times high risk of heart failure compared with those without diabetes.

Attributable risk

In the discussion above, the measures of risk difference and RR are applied to estimate the strength of an association between an exposure and risk of disease. A further question is how much of the disease that occurs can be attributable to a particular exposure? In other words, how much of the risk of disease can we hope to prevent if we can eliminate the exposure in question? That is, we want to quantify the possible consequences of exposure to a risk factor for a population. To answer this question, we need to calculate *attributable risks* (*AR*). It has an important meaning in healthcare planning and health education because it emphasizes the possibility of the disease that could be prevented if we eliminate the exposure. By estimating the extent to which a disease is related to a particular risk factor, healthcare planners can predict the effectiveness of control or prevention programs.

Example. To calculate AR using data from Table 4.5

$$AR = (\text{Disease risk in exposed group})$$
$$- (\text{Disease risk in non-exposed group})$$
$$= 17.5 - 10.83$$
$$= 6.67 \ (\text{‰})$$

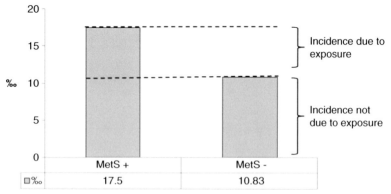

FIG. 4.4 Hypothetical data to calculate attributable risk.

Interpretation: The risk of incident heart failure is increased by 6.67‰ for those individuals who exposure to MetS. Fig. 4.4 depicts the risk difference.

In practice, we also estimate a measure called the attributable risk percent (AR%, or called attributable proportion or the etiologic fraction). AR% answers what the proportion of the risk of disease in the exposed group is due to the exposure.

$$AR\% = \frac{(\text{Incidence in exposure group} - \text{incidence in non-exposure group})}{\text{Incidence in expsoure group}} \times 100$$
$$= (17.5 - 10.83)/17.5 \times 100$$
$$= 38.11\ (\%)$$

The results suggest that 38.11% of the incidence of heart failure were attributable to MetS among the MetS group. That 38.11% of the incident heart failure could presumably be prevented by eliminating MetS.

Population attributable risk (PAR)

AR answers how much the risk of disease due to the exposure among exposed group. In risk assessment at a population level, we may further want to know much the risk of disease due to the exposure in the total population. We then calculate PAR.

$$PAR = \text{Incidence in total population incidence} \\ \text{in non-exposed group}$$

Example. To calculate PAR using data from Table 4.5

$$PAR = 12.5 - 10.83$$
$$= 1.67\ (\%)$$

Interpretation: the excess incidence (i.e., risk) of heart failure in the total study population that is associated with MetS is 1.67 per 1000 population.

Similar to AR percent, we can calculate PAR percent (PAR%).

$$PAR\% = \frac{(\text{Incidence in total population-incidence in non-expsoure group})}{\text{Incidence in total populaiton}} \times 100$$
$$PAR\% = (12.5 - 10.83)/12.5 \times 100$$
$$= 13.36\ \%$$

Interpretation: In the hypothetical data, 13.36% of the excess incidence in the total population is attributable to MetS, and if an effective prevention program could eliminate MetS, the best that we expected to achieve would be a reduction of 13.36% in the incidence of heart failure in the total population.

Application of relative risk and attributable risk

RR is a measure of the strength of the association between an exposure and disease. It provides evidence that can be used to judge whether a strong observed association is likely to be causal.

AR is a measure of the impact of exposure on the public health, assuming that the association between an exposure and a particular disease is one of the cause and effect.

Population attributable risk (PAR) is a measure of the reduction in incidence (or an estimate of prevalence or mortality) that would be observed if the population were entirely unexposed, compared with its current (actual) exposure pattern. This concept was first proposed by Levin in 1953 and is widely used in epidemiologic studies and health education programs.[7,8]

Hazard ratio

In survival analysis, the hazard ratio is the ratio of the hazard rates corresponding to the conditions described by two levels of an explanatory variable. For example, in a heart failure outcome study, patients with heart failure may have two times higher risk of death than those without heart failure. We will discuss this in more detail in Chapter 5.

ANALYTICAL BIOSTATISTICS (I)

Definition of Analytical Biostatistics

Analytical biostatistics targets more statistical concepts of inferential statistics. It includes testing of hypothesis, distribution of data and theory of estimation, sample size, power analysis, and predictive modeling.

Basic Concepts

Population and sample

The population is the whole collection of units from which a sample may be drawn. A sample is a subset of the population, selected so as to be representative of the population. The sample is intended to yield results that are representative of the entire population.

Because it is often not feasible or even not necessary to collect information on all objects in a population, we then select participants from the total population. The selected participants are a sample of the total population and with an assumption of a representative sample of the entire population in which they are selected.

Example: if we are interested in estimating mean SBP in adults aged 45 and older who are living in the state of Pennsylvania, theoretically, we could recruit all residents aged 45 and older and measure and calculate the mean SBP in the state of Pennsylvania. However, practically, we often select a sample (say, randomly select 1000 residents aged 45 and older), then measure their SBP, and get the mean $(\overline{X})$ SBP from the selected participants. Our purpose is to use the mean value $(\overline{X})$ from the sample data (i.e., 1000 residents) to estimate the total mean (μ) in the entire residents aged 45 and older in the state of Pennsylvania. In biostatistics, the entire residents aged 45 and older in the state of Pennsylvania is the population, and the selected participants (i.e., 1000) is a sample.

Parameter and statistic

In biostatistics, a parameter is a value or characteristic associated with a population, such as population mean (noted as μ) and population SD (noted as σ). A statistic is a value or characteristic calculated from a sample,

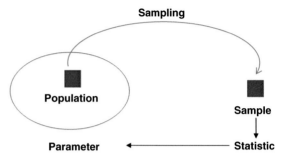

FIG. 4.5 Randomly select parts of observations from the total population to get a sample. From the sample to calculate a statistic (such as mean), for the purpose of estimating the parameter (such as mean) of the total population.

such as a sample mean (noted as $\overline{X}$) and sample standard deviation (noted as SD). We are always interested in estimating population values (i.e., parameters) from samples (i.e., statistics) (Fig. 4.5).

Methods of sampling

Sampling is a process used in biostatistics analysis in which a predetermined number of observations are taken from a larger population. A random, or probability, sample is selected from the target or study population that an investigator hopes to study. Selecting a random sample requires choosing a representative group of the members of a population in a way that ensures each member is independently chosen and has a known chance (i.e., nonzero probability) of being selected.

The methodology used to sample from a larger population depends on the type of analysis being performed. It includes four common methods. (1) Simple random sampling: It is one in which everyone has an equal probability of being selected for the study. (2) Systematic sampling: It is the procedure of selecting according to some simple, systematic rule, such as all persons whose names begin with specified alphabetic letters, born on certain dates, etc., on a master list. (3) Stratified sampling: It is one in which the population is first divided into relevant strata (subgroups), and a random sample is then selected from each stratum. (4) Cluster sampling: It is a two-stage process in which the population is divided into clusters (e.g., neighborhood) and a subset of the clusters is randomly selected.[2]

Sampling error

In the above example, if we reselect 1000 residents aged 45 and older from the same total residents, we use the same sampling method (i.e., simple randomly selection); the mean SBP from the second sample is likely to close to the first selected sample, but it is unlikely to be exactly equal. The same would be that even more repeated samples were selected and compared. Certainly, the mean from a sampling is not exactly equal to the total population mean. The difference in the means between the sample and the total population is called sampling error because this difference results from the sampling. That sampling error occurs because only a sample of the population is investigated. To minimize a sampling error, one can increase the sample size of the selection (such as increase the sample size to 10,000, or more) and make sure the sampling selection approaches are correct and standardized.

Sampling distribution
It is essential to understand sampling distribution for grasping the logic underlying the prototypical statistical statements from the literature. It helps us to understand and learn about estimation and hypothesis testing, the methods that permit investigators to generalize study results to the population that the sample represents. Fig. 4.6 depicts the frequency distributions of SBP in a study sample. Fig. 4.6A depicts when the sample size is 2913, the mean of SBP = 137.9 mm Hg, SD = 21.2. Fig. 4.6B depicts when a random sample (n = 1000) is selected from 2913, the mean of SBP = 137.2 mm Hg, SD = 20.9. Fig. 4.6C depicts when a random sample (n = 50) is selected from 2913, the mean of SBP = 136.6 mm Hg, SD = 19.4. All three figures are in an approximately bell-shaped distribution, although Fig. 4.6A and B shows more similarity. If we assume that Fig. 4.6A represents the "total population," when a subsample is selected from the "total population," the means of SBP from the subsample would be not equal to the "total population" mean, such as Fig. 4.6B and C. The frequency distribution of SBP in a subsample with a larger sample size (such as, N = 1000) is closer to the distribution of SBP in the "total population" than that in a subsample with a smaller sample size (i.e., N = 50). It suggests that an appropriate sample size is important to estimate parameters in a population of interest.

Standard error of mean: the standard deviation of mean
As we discussed earlier, in the real world, we have a sample dataset from a target population and we are using the sample statistic (such as sample mean) to estimate the population parameter (i.e., population

mean). However, a sample mean is a point estimator of the population mean. To estimate the difference between the means, an investigator could conduct the sampling survey many times (i.e., samples 1, 2, 3, … χ), calculate their means, and then quantify this variability by measuring the SD of the means. The SD of the mean is called the standard error of the mean. The distribution of means is called the sampling distribution of the mean.

It should be noted that the properties of the sampling distribution of mean are the basis for one of the most important theorems in statistics, called central limit theorem. The properties are as follows. (1) The mean of the sampling distribution, or the mean of the means, is equal to the population mean (μ) based on the individual observations. (2) The SD of the sampling distribution of the mean (i.e., standard error of the mean, SEM) is equal to $\sigma/\sqrt{n}$, where σ is the population SD. This quantity of SEM plays an important role in many statistical tests.

$$SEM = \sigma/\sqrt{n}$$

In most cases, we can calculate the SD from a sample; then we can estimate the SEM using the following formula.

$$\text{Estimated SEM} = SD/\sqrt{n}$$

Example. To estimate the SEM from the sample means of SBP:

N1 = 2931, SD = 21.22
N2 = 1000, SD = 20.9
N3 = 50, SD = 19.4

$$SEM \text{ of sample 1 } (N = 2931) = 21.22/\sqrt{2931}$$
$$= 21.22/54.14$$
$$= 0.39$$

$$SEM \text{ of sample 2 } (N = 1000) = 20.9/\sqrt{1000}$$
$$= 20.9/31.62$$
$$= 0.66$$

$$SEM \text{ of sample 3 } (N = 50) = 19.4/\sqrt{50}$$
$$= 19.4/7.07$$
$$= 2.74$$

A larger SEM indicates greater sampling error. It is clear that increase in sample size can decrease sampling error.

Standard deviation versus standard error of mean
In Descriptive Biostatistics section, we discussed SD. The value of SD in the population (σ) or a sample (SD) is based on measures of individuals. SDs tell

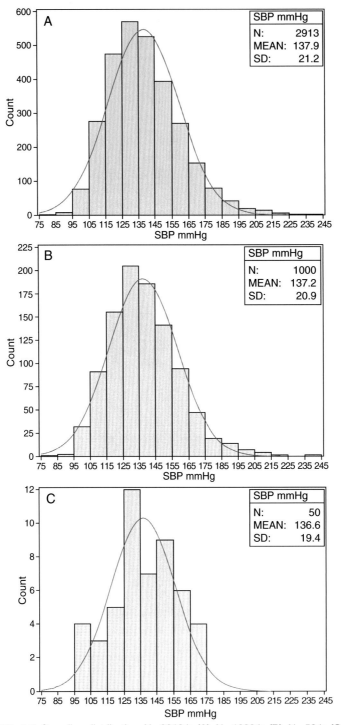

FIG. 4.6 Sampling distribution: N = 2913 in **(A)**, N = 1000 in **(B)**, N = 50 in **(C)**.

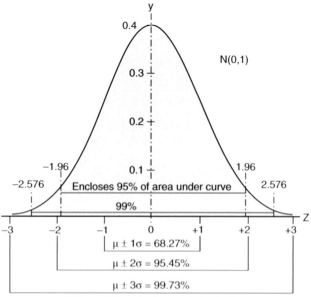

FIG. 4.7 Standard normal distribution.

us how much variability can be expected among individuals.

The SEM, however, is the SD of the means in a sampling distribution of the means; it tells us how much variability can be expected among means in future samples.

The sampling distribution of the mean is applied (1) to estimate confidence intervals (CIs) and (2) to conduct hypothesis testing. Their applications are based on a normal distribution theory.

Normal Distribution

A symmetrical bell-shaped distribution is called normal distribution (also called Gaussian distribution). It is defined by two parameters: mean and SD. There are three key features of a normal distribution. (1) It is a continuous symmetrical distribution; both tails extend to infinity. (2) The arithmetic mean, mode, and median are identical. (3) Its shape is completely determined by the mean and SD.

Standard normal distribution

A standard normal distribution is a normal distribution with a mean of zero and an SD of one. It is often called the bell curve (or z distribution) because the graph of its probability density resembles a bell (Fig. 4.7). Areas under portions of the standard normal distribution ($\mu = 0$, and $\sigma = 1$) are shown in the figure. About 0.95 of the distribution is between −1.96 and 1.96; and about 0.99 of the distribution is between −2.58 and 2.58.

The standard normal distribution is a fundamental that is applied in percentile CI estimate and hypothesis testing, although data from the real world is never exactly shaped in the way of a standard normal distribution.

Confidence intervals for population mean (μ)

As previously discussed, it is usually not possible to have population parameters directly (such as population mean, μ). Instead, the value of the parameter is estimated by the corresponding sample statistic (sample mean, $\bar{X}$). Because the value of the sample statistic varies from sample to sample (as measured by the SEM), uncertainty is introduced into this estimation process. However, if the population parameter (such as μ) and a sample from the population have a normal distribution, we can apply the standard normal distribution theory (the areas under proportions) to estimate a percentile of the CI of the population parameter (such as 95%CI). The CI method of estimating a population parameter takes into account of the sample to sample variation of the statistic by defining an interval within which the true population parameter is likely to fall. Fig. 4.8 depicts the calculation of a 95%CI of mean. The lower end of the CI (estimate − 1.96 * SEM) is called the lower confidence limit (LCL). The upper end of the CI (estimate + 1.96 * SEM) is called the upper confidence limit (UCL).

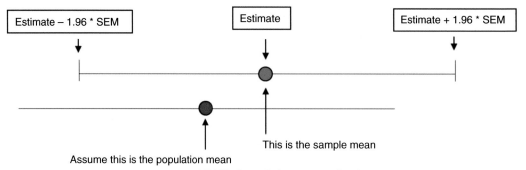

FIG. 4.8 95%CI of population mean estimation.

The length of the CI (=UCL−LCL) quantifies the precision of the estimate. Short CIs suggest that the sample estimate is quite precise and provide a reasonably good estimate of the population mean. Long CIs suggest that the estimate is relatively imprecise.

Example. We can calculate their 95%CI of means using the same dataset in Fig. 4.6, samples A, B, and C.

In sample A, N = 2931, mean SBP = 137.86, and SEM = 0.39. The mean SBP (=137.86 mm Hg) computed from the sample of 2913 provides a point estimate of the mean SBP level of the total targeted population. Our further interest is what the 95%CI is. The calculation is shown below.

$$95\%CI \text{ of the mean} = 137.86 \pm 1.96 * 0.39$$
$$= 137.07 \sim 138.63$$

Interpretation, the investigator may have 95% confidence that the mean SBP in the population of residents who are aged 45 years and older lies within the interval between 137.07 mm Hg and 136.63 mm Hg.

The same as the above, we can estimate the 95%CI of means for samples B and C.

$$\text{In sample B, N} = 1000, \text{ mean SBP} = 137.24, \text{ and}$$
$$\text{SEM} = 0.66, \text{ then}$$
$$95\%CI \text{ of the mean} = 137.24 \pm 1.96 * 0.66$$
$$= 135.95 \sim 138.54$$

$$\text{In sample C, N} = 50, \text{ mean SBP} = 136.62, \text{ and}$$
$$\text{SEM} = 2.74, \text{ then}$$
$$95\%CI \text{ of the mean} = 136.62 \pm 1.96 * 2.74$$
$$= 131.12 \sim 142.12$$

In sample C, it has a wider CI than the others. It suggests that the mean estimate (136.62) from a sample size of 50 is relatively imprecise.

In the discussion above, a CI estimate is based on the distribution of the variable of interest. If a study variable of interest is not distributed normally, the 95%CI estimate approach is incorrect. In the situation, a data transformation step may be considered. The most commonly used transformation is log transformation.

Example. In the same dataset, HFBKBG 1, serum mean triglycerides (TG) = 148.56 mg/dL, SD = 76.53, SEM = 1.55. Fig. 4.9A depicts the distribution of TG (mg/dL). It is not in a normal distribution. Therefore, to estimate the mean value and its 95%CI should be done by transforming TG into a normal distribution. Fig. 4.9B depicts the distribution of log-TG is in an approximately normal distribution.

Methods for Data Transformation
Several methods have been suggested to transfer data with nonnormal distribution to a normal or an approximately normal distribution.[2]

Logarithms
Growth rates are often exponential and log transforms will often normalize them. Log transforms are particularly appropriate if the variance increases with the mean.

Reciprocal (inverse)
If a log transform does not normalize the data of interest, we may try a reciprocal (1/x) transformation. This is often used for enzyme reaction rate data.

Square root
This transform is often of value when the data are counts, e.g., blood cells on a hemocytometer or woodlice in a garden. Carrying out a square root transform will convert data with a Poisson distribution to a normal distribution.

Serum TG level, mg/dL

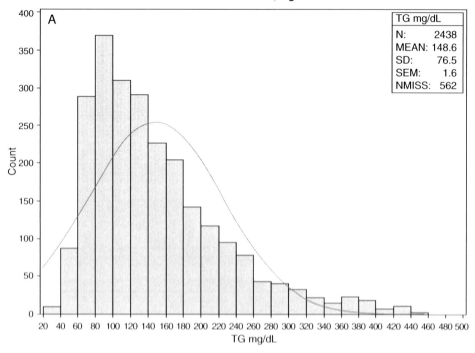

Log-transformed serum TG level, mg/dL

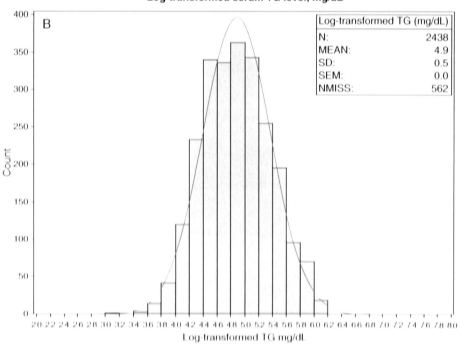

FIG. 4.9 Sampling distributions: Serum triglycerides mg/dL **(A)**, and Log-transformed values of triglycerides mg/dL **(B)**.

Arcsine

This transformation is also known as the angular transformation and is especially useful for percentages and proportions.

Parametric data versus nonparametric data

In biostatistics, data in a normal or an approximately normal distribution is called as parametric data. For this type of data, parametric analysis methods are requested in hypothesis testing. It is clear what we have discussed conference intervals are based on the data in a normal distribution.

Data in a nonnormal or not approximately normal distribution are called as nonparametric data. For this type of data, nonparametric analysis methods are requested in hypothesis testing, and an estimation of the "conference interval" is not recommended.

SAS Computing

To estimate the standard error of mean SBP and 95%CI of mean using data, HFBKBG1:

SAS Proc step

```
PROC MEANS N MEAN STD STDERR CLM CV MIN MAX NMISS MAXDEC=2 DATA=HFBKBG1;
VAR SBP;
TITLE 'N= 2913';
RUN;
```

Output

				N= 2913					
				The MEANS Procedure					
				Analysis Variable : sbp SBP mmHg					
N	Mean	Std Dev	Std Error	Lower 95% CL for Mean	Upper 95% CL for Mean	Coeff of Variation	Minimum	Maximum	N Miss
2913	137.86	21.22	0.39	137.09	138.63	15.39	81.00	244.00	87

The results indicate that mean SBP = 137.88, SD = 21.22, SEM = 0.39, and 95%CI = 137.09 ~ 138.63. Of total dataset (N = 3000), there were 87 with missing values of SBP, leave the calculation sample size of 2913.

To describe the distribution, we apply SAS univariate procedure.

SAS Proc step

```
PROC UNIVARIATE DATA = HFBKBG1;
VAR SBP;
HISTOGRAM SBP / NORMAL VSCALE = COUNT CFILL = grey ENDPOINTS=(75 TO 250 BY 10);
INSET N='N:' (5.0) MEAN='MEAN:' (6.1) STD='SD:' (6.1)/
HEADER = 'SBP mmHg' CFILL = WHITE POS =NE HEIGHT=2;
RUN;
```

To get log-transform TG in Data step, the data statement as below.

```
DATA HFBKBG2;
SET HFBKBG1;
LOG_TG = LOG (TG);

LABEL
TG ='TG mg/dL'
LOG_TG ='Log-transformed TG mg/dL'
;
RUN;
```

To describe the distribution of log-transformed TG:
SAS Proc step

```
PROC UNIVARIATE DATA = HFBKBG2;
VAR LOG_TG;
HISTOGRAM LOG_TG / NORMAL VSCALE = COUNT CFILL = grey   ENDPOINTS = (2 TO 8 BY 0.2);
INSET N='N:' (5.0) MEAN='MEAN:' (6.1) STD='SD:' (6.1) STDERR='SEM:' (6.1) nmiss='NMISS:' /
HEADER = 'Log-transformed TG (mg/dL)' CFILL = WHITE POS =NE HEIGHT=2;
TITLE 'Log-transformed serum TG level, mg/dL';
RUN;
```

Output: see Fig. 4.9B.

ANALYTICAL BIOSTATISTICS (II)

Analytical biostatistics is also called inferential statistics. It is applied to make generalizations or "inferences" about a large group or population using information derived from a representative sample of the study population of interest.

In medical research, whether it involves testing a relationship between biomarker and risk of diseases, such as heart failure, or a relationship between a new drug use and risk reduction of heart failure, it begins with a research question (or questions). This research question is typically posed as a research hypothesis, postulating the existence of a difference between groups or an association among risk (or protective) factors. To answer this question, data are obtained from a sample or samples drawn from the populations of interest. However, because of random variation, even an unbiased sample may not accurately represent the population as a whole. As a result, it is possible that any observed differences between groups or associations between variables may have occurred by chance. The intent of an inferential statistical test is to determine whether there is enough evidence to "reject" a conjecture or hypothesis about the existence of an association or difference. It is what we call "significance test"—the process used by investigators to determine whether a "no difference" or "no association" (i.e., the null hypothesis) is rejected or in favor of the existence of an association or difference (i.e., the alternative hypothesis).

Basic Steps in a Hypothesis Testing
Step 1: set up null and alternative hypotheses
To convert a research question into null hypothesis (H_0) and an alternative hypothesis (H_1), for example, we test the differences in means of SBP between subjects with or without heart failure.

Example. Null hypothesis (H_0) is a statement of "no difference" in means of SBP ($\mu_1 = \mu_2$, or $\mu_1 - \mu_2 = 0$) between the two study populations. They can be noted as below.

$$H_0: \mu_1 = \mu_2 \text{ or, } \mu_1 - \mu_2 = 0$$

The opposing hypothesis is the alternative hypothesis (H_1). It is a statement of "there is a difference" (H_1: $\mu_1 \neq \mu_2$ or, $\mu_1 - \mu_2 \neq 0$) in means of SBP between the two study populations.

$$H_1: \mu_1 = \mu_2 \text{ or, } \mu_1 - \mu_2 = 0$$

In sampling studies, we test differences in sample mean ($\bar{X}$).

For example, to test the mean SBP difference between those with and without heart failure, the null hypothesis (H_0) states that there are no differences. If the null hypothesis is rejected, we then accept the alternative hypothesis (i.e., there are differences in mean SBP between the two study populations).

Step 2: select significance level
How much difference between the comparison of interest (such as means SPB between subjects with and without heart failure) is the reject level or the acceptable level of a null hypothesis? In biostatistics, we select a significance level. Fig. 4.10 depicts the basic concept of

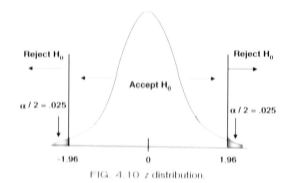

FIG. 4.10 z distribution.

a significance level selection using z-test as an example to explain the selection of significance level.

Definition of z-test

A z-test is a statistical test used to determine whether two population means are different when the variances are known, and the sample size is large. The test statistic is assumed to have a normal distribution (with mean, $\mu = 0$ and SD = 1), and nuisance parameters such as SD should be known for an accurate **z-test** to be performed.

$$Z - \text{test is defined as } z = (\bar{X} - \mu)/ \left(\sigma/\sqrt{n} \right)$$

where $\bar{x}$ is the sample mean, μ is the population mean, σ in the population SD, n is the population sample size, and $(\sigma/\sqrt{n})$ is the population SD of mean (SEM).

In the formula above, a population mean should be from a population with a normal distribution or for any sample with large sample size n for which the sample mean will follow a normal distribution by the central limit theorem. If the SD σ is known, the appropriate significance test is known.

The areas under the whole portion of z distribution (normal distribution) are 100% (can be considered as probability). If a z-score is between > -1.96 and < 1.96, it will fall within the areas of ± 1 SD (i.e., 95% probabilities). In null hypothesis, we assume that a sample mean $(\bar{X})$ is from the total population, that the value of $\bar{x}$ should be closer to the population mean (μ). However, if the sample mean has a huge difference from the population mean, a large z-score (absolute value) will be obtained from the z-score formula. If the estimated z-score is ≤ -1.96 or ≥ 1.96, the probability of having this value is less than$\leq 5\%$ ($P \leq .05$, the two sides combined in the tails of Fig. 4.10). In the situation (i.e., $P \leq .05$), we reject the null hypothesis and accept the alternative hypothesis in which the sample mean is significantly different from the total population mean.

In a hypothesis testing, the values used frequently for significance levels are 0.05 and 0.01:
- When P-value $> .05$, the observed difference is not significant (i.e., accept H_0).
- When P-value $\leq .05$, the observed difference is significant (i.e., reject H_0).
- When P-value $\leq .01$, the observed difference is highly significant (i.e., reject H_0).

For z-test (i.e., data with a normal distribution):

Estimated z Statistic	P-value	Significance	H_0
> -1.96 and < 1.96	$> .05$	No	Accept
$\geq \lvert 1.96 \rvert$ and $< \lvert 2.58 \rvert$	$\leq .05$	Yes	Reject
$\geq \lvert 2.58 \rvert$	≤ 01	Yes	Reject

Two-tailed or one-tailed test

Another important concept in significance testing is whether we use a one-tailed or two-tailed test of significance.

The answer is that it depends on our hypothesis. When our research hypothesis states the direction of the difference or relationship, then we use a one-tailed probability. For example, a one-tailed test may be used to test this null hypothesis: serum 25-hydroxyvitamin D concentration in heart failure patients will be not lower than heart failure without chronic kidney disease. In the case, the null hypothesis predicts the direction of the difference.

On the other hand, a two-tailed test would be used to test this null hypothesis: There is no significant difference in serum 25-hydroxyvitamin D concentration between heart failure patients with or without chronic kidney disease. In the case, the direction of comparison (lower or higher) is not specified. Fig. 4.10 shows standard z distribution, when $z = 1.96$, the P-value $= .05$ (if for a two-tailed test, P-value $= .025 + 0.025 = 0.05$).

Step 3: select an appropriate statistic

There are different types of test statistics for various situations. The test statistic is based on the specific hypothesis to be tested and the types of data for the key variables of interest (i.e., a continuous or categorical or ordinal variable). For example, to test a difference between two means (continuous variables), we may use z-test (if sample size $>= 30$) or t-test (if sample size < 30). To test differences among three or more means, we should use analysis of variation (ANOVA), instead of the t-test.

Step 4: calculate the selected statistic and conclusion

This step is to calculate a statistic, to get P-value, and then to get a conclusion on whether to reject a null hypothesis or accept the alternative hypothesis based on a predecided significance level (i.e., commonly, $P \leq .05$ or ≤ 0.01).

z-Test for Comparing Two Means

Data requirements: The comparable variables from each of the two sample datasets are in a normal distribution.

Step 1: Hypotheses

Null hypothesis (H0): $\bar{X}_1 - \bar{X}_2 = \mu = 0$

Alternative hypothesis (H1): $\bar{X}_1 - \bar{X}_2 \neq \mu \neq 0$

Step 2: Select significance level: $P \leq .05$

Step 3: Select statistic

$$z = \frac{\bar{x}_1 - \bar{x}_2 - \Delta}{\sqrt{\dfrac{\sigma_1^2}{n_1} + \dfrac{\sigma_2^2}{n_2}}}$$

TABLE 4.6
Example of z-Test Comparing Two Means

	HF	No.	SBP MM HG Mean	SD
People without HF	No	2787	137.6	21.11
People with HF	Yes	213	141.6	22.26
z-test				
Δ			0	
Mean 1 – Mean 2 – Δ (a)			–3.99	
SD_1^2/n_1 (b)			0.16	
SD_2^2/n_2 (c)			2.33	
Square root of (b + c) (d)			1.58	
z score = (a)/(d)			–2.53	

HF, heart failure.

where $\bar{x}_1$ and $\bar{x}_2$ are the means of the two samples, Δ is the hypothesized difference between the population means (0 if testing for equal means), σ_1 and σ_2 are the SDs of the two populations, and n_1 and n_2 are the sizes of the two samples.

Example

This example is to compare two sample means SBP (mm Hg), one in subjects without heart failure (HF), n = 2787, mean SBP = 137.6 mm Hg, SD = 21.11, and the other sample in patients with HF, n = 213, SBP = 141.6 mm Hg, SD = 22.26 (Table 4.6). Because the total population deviations in two samples are not available, we apply the two samples' SDs as the estimates.

Table 4.6 shows the data and calculation. The result indicates that z-score = –2.53, which is more than |1.96|, but less than |2.58|, then we reject the null hypothesis at *P* value <.05. In conclusion, patients with heart failure have significantly higher SBP than those without heart failure.

$$z = \frac{\bar{x}_1 - \bar{x}_2 - \Delta}{\sqrt{\frac{\sigma_1^2}{n_1} + \frac{\sigma_2^2}{n_2}}}$$
$$= |137.6 - 141.6 - 0|/\sqrt{1.58}$$
$$= 2.53$$

t-Test for Comparing Two Means

Most people may be familiar with the name "Student" but not with the name Gosset. In fact, Gosset wrote under the name "Student," which explains why his

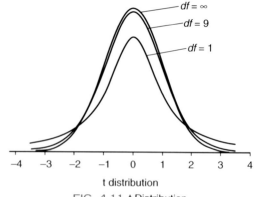
FIG. 4.11 t Distribution.

name may be less known than his important results in statistics. He invented the t-test to handle small samples for quality control in brewing.[1,9]

t distribution

We know the standard normal distribution, or z distribution, is symmetric with a mean of 0 and SD of 1. The t distribution is also symmetric and has a mean of 0, but its SD is large than 1. The precise size of the SD depends on a complex concept related to the sample size, called degrees of freedom (df). It refers the number of times sample information is used. For example, the t distribution for one group has n–1 degrees of freedom, because the sample information is used only once to estimate the SD.

When the sample size is small (say, <30), the t distribution has a larger SD; its trials are higher than those for the z distribution. However, as the sample size increases to 30 or more (i.e., the degrees of freedom increase), the t distribution becomes almost the same as the standard normal distribution. Fig. 4.11 shows t distribution with df = 1, df = 9, and df = infinity. Understanding this is important, because (1) we assume that the observations (factors) of interest are normally distributed, we then use t test for a comparison between two means. (2) t test is used when sample sizes are small (i.e., <30). When the compared factors from two large sample datasets, we can either use z test or t test, because t distribution is closer to a normal distribution when its sample size increases.

Two most common t tests are applied: (1) paired t test for mean difference, and (2) nonpaired t test for two independent samples.

Paired t-test for mean difference from one group of samples

Paired sample t test compares means where the two groups are correlated, such as data from the same

TABLE 4.7
Example for Paired t Test

ID	BMI, KG/M^2 WEEK0	WEEK12	DIFF
1	35	37	–2
2	32	26	6
3	27	28	–1
4	26	24	2
5	33	27	6
6	28	26	2
7	26	23	3
8	28	27	1
9	33	27	6
10	30	24	6
Mean	29.8	26.9	2.9
SD	3.26	3.9	3.03

participants before-and-after, or repeated measures, matched-pairs, or case-control studies (e.g., left ventricular ejection fractions are measured before and after an intervention). The algorithm applied to the data using paired t-test is different from the independent sample t-test, but the interpretation of output is otherwise the same.

$$\text{Paired } t = (\overline{X}_d - 0) / (SD_d/\sqrt{n})$$

where $\overline{X}_d$ stands for the mean difference and $(SD_d/\sqrt{n})$ is the standard error of the mean difference.

Example. Table 4.7 shows an intensive intervention program for 10 subjects with BMI more than 25 kg/m^2. After a 12-week lifestyle change (diet and physical activity) trial, BMIs are compared between baseline and at week 12. Paired t-test is applied to test the mean difference in subjects with before and after the intervention.

$$\text{Paired } t = (2.90 - 0) / (3.03/\sqrt{10})$$
$$= 3.04$$

Please note, because t distribution is changed with the number of observation (or degree of freedom, df), when t statistic is calculated, it should be compared with the t values in a standard t-distribution table. In the example, n = 10, df = 10 − 1 = 9, from t-distribution table (Table 4.8), when df = 9, if P-value = .05 (for two-tailed test), t-value = 2.26; and if P-value = .01 (for two-tailed test), t-value = 3.25. That is, our observed t-value (3.04)

>2.26, $P<.05$. We reject the null hypothesis. In other words, the mean difference in BMI between baseline and after a 12-week intervention is significant ($P<.05$).

t-Test for two independent means

When comparing two means from two separate populations or samples (such as comparing mean SBP in those with or without heart failure), we may use independent samples t-test.

$$\text{Independent samples } t-\text{test} = (\overline{X}_1 - \overline{X}_2)/SE_{1-2}$$

where $\overline{X}_1$ is the mean of interest in sample 1, $\overline{X}_2$ is the mean of interest in sample 2, and SE_{1-2} is the standard error of the mean difference.

$$SE_{1-2} = \sqrt{\frac{S1^2}{n1} + \frac{S2^2}{n2}}$$

where $S1^2$ and n1 are the SDs in sample 1 and $S2^2$ and n2 are the SD in sample 2.

Example. In a study, compare mean age in two samples: one in subjects without heart failure (HF), n = 2787, mean age = 66.65 years, SD = 12.29 and the other sample in patients with HF, n = 213, mean age = 71.05, SD = 10.52. Our research question is whether the mean ages are significant between the two samples. We may use the t-test for two independent samples.

$$t = (66.65 - 71.05) \div \sqrt{(12.29^2 \div 2787) + (10.52^2 \div 213)}$$
$$= -6.23$$

Because the sample size is big enough (more than 1000), we can either look at t distribution table or use u-test values for a normal distribution data. The estimated absolute t value = |6.23| > 2.58; therefore the two sample mean ages have highly significant differences ($P<.01$).

Analysis of Variance for Comparing Three or More than Three Means

Research question: In HFKBBG1 dataset, participants smoking status are categorized into three groups, never smoking (n = 1948), formerly smoked (n = 278), and current smokers (774). The mean (SD) ages are 67.16 (12.65), 67.41 (10.92), and 62.72 (11.02), for never smoking, formerly smoked, and current smokers, respectively. One of the research questions is whether the mean ages are significantly different by three smoking status. As it is to test mean differences across three groups, one-way analysis of variance (ANOVA) test can be used.

We can consider one-way ANOVA as an extension of the t-tests that we have described in independent sample t-test for two means. However, when a

TABLE 4.8
t-Distribution Table With One- and Two-Tail Probabilities in Selected Degree of Freedom (DF)

One Tail: Significant Level α							
0.0005	0.001	0.005	0.01	0.02	0.025	0.05	0.1

Two Tails: Significant Level α							
DF	0.001	0.002	0.01	0.02	0.04	0.05	0.1	0.2
1	636.6192	318.3088	63.6567	31.8205	15.8945	12.7062	6.3138	3.0777
2	31.5991	22.3271	9.9248	6.9646	4.8487	4.3027	2.9200	1.8856
3	12.9240	10.2145	5.8409	4.5407	3.4819	3.1824	2.3534	1.6377
4	8.6103	7.1732	4.6041	3.7469	2.9985	2.7764	2.1318	1.5332
5	6.8688	5.8934	4.0321	3.3649	2.7565	2.5706	2.0150	1.4759
6	5.9588	5.2076	3.7074	3.1427	2.6122	2.4469	1.9432	1.4398
7	5.4079	4.7853	3.4995	2.9980	2.5168	2.3646	1.8946	1.4149
8	5.0413	4.5008	3.3554	2.8965	2.4490	2.3060	1.8595	1.3968
9	4.7809	4.2968	3.2498	2.8214	2.3984	2.2622	1.8331	1.3830
10	4.5869	4.1437	3.1693	2.7638	2.3593	2.2281	1.8125	1.3722
15	4.0728	3.7328	2.9467	2.6025	2.2485	2.1314	1.7531	1.3406
20	3.8495	3.5518	2.8453	2.5280	2.1967	2.0860	1.7247	1.3253
25	3.7251	3.4502	2.7874	2.4851	2.1666	2.0595	1.7081	1.3163
30	3.6460	3.3852	2.7500	2.4573	2.1470	2.0423	1.6973	1.3104
35	3.5911	3.3400	2.7238	2.4377	2.1332	2.0301	1.6896	1.3062
70	3.4350	3.2108	2.6479	2.3808	2.0927	1.9944	1.6669	1.2938
80	3.4163	3.1953	2.6387	2.3739	2.0878	1.9901	1.6641	1.2922
90	3.4019	3.1833	2.6316	2.3685	2.0839	1.9867	1.6620	1.2910
100	3.3905	3.1737	2.6259	2.3642	2.0809	1.9840	1.6602	1.2901
120	3.3735	3.1595	2.6174	2.3578	2.0763	1.9799	1.6577	1.2886
1,000,000	3.2905	3.0902	2.5758	2.3264	2.0538	1.9600	1.6449	1.2816

Example: To determine the 0.05 critical value (two tails) from the t-distribution with 9 degrees of freedom, look in the 0.05 column at the 9 row: t(0.05,9) = 2.2622.

hypothesis testing for three or more means significance test, ANOVA test should be used, but not t test.

The basic concept of ANOVA test, as its name suggests, focuses on the variabilities of the factors (continuous variables, such as age in the example) between the groups of interests (such as smoking status in the example) and variabilities of the factors among individuals within each group. The result of this calculation is expressed using a statistic called the F ratio (writing simply as F). The mathematical formulas are little complicated. Fortunately, a standard software can conduct the analysis in few seconds. The table below is the main result of testing a null hypothesis that the three population means of age across smoking status (never, former and current smokers) are equal. The calculation is done using SAS Proc ANOVA.

Source	DF	Sum of Squares	Mean Square	F Value	P > F
Model	2	11,502.9954	5751.4977	39.40	< .0001
Error	2997	438,566.4683	146.3352		
Corrected Total	2999	450,069.4637			

R-Square	Coeff Var	Root MSE	Age Mean
0.025558	18.31912	12.09691	66.03433

Output: The table below shows the overall testing; F value = 39.30 and $P < .0001$. It suggests that means of age are significantly different across three smoking status.

Source	DF	Anova SS	Mean Square	F Value	P > F
smk	2	11,502.99538	5751.49769	39.30	<.0001

Output: The table below shows the mean comparisons. It indicates that the differences in mean age between current smokers (62.72) and former smokers (67.41, age difference = 4.67), and between never smokers (67.16) and current smokers (age difference = 4.44), are statistically significant at a P-value of 0.05 level (indicated by ***).

Comparisons Significant at the 0.05 Level are Indicated by***

SMK Comparison	Difference Between Means	Simultaneous 95% Confidence Limits		
FORMER—NO	0.2494	−1.5692	2.0680	
FORMER—CURRENT	4.6907	2.7073	6.6741	***
NO—FORMER	−0.2494	−2.0680	1.5692	
NO—CURRENT	4.4413	3.2361	5.6466	***
CURRENT—FORMER	−4.6907	−6.6741	−2.7073	***
CURRENT—NO	−4.4413	−5.6466	−3.2361	***

The ANOVA Procedure

Level of SMK	N	Age	
		Mean	Std Dev
CURRENT	774	62.7157623	11.0157753
FORMER	278	67.4064748	10.9216224
NO	1948	67.1570842	12.6532502

When conducting ANOVA test, the data tested should meet three basic assumptions.

1. The values of the dependent (or outcome) variables (for example, SBP) are assumed to be normally distributed within each group or level of the factor.
2. The population variance is the same in each group. In practice, we may look at whether SDs of each group are approximately equal. (Rule of thumb: ratio of largest to smallest sample SD must be less than 2:1.)
3. The observations are a random sample, and they are independent in that the value of one observation is not related in any way to the value of another observation.

If a dataset does not meet the assumptions, a non-parametric analysis should be conducted to test the differences in mean across the groups of interests.

Nonparametric Tests

Nonparametric tests are used in detecting population differences when certain assumptions are not satisfied.

Wilcoxon signed rank test

Wilcoxon signed rank test, a rank test used in non-parametric statistics, can be considered as a backup for t-test where the independent variable is binary but the dependent variable is not normally distributed. It is used to compare the locations of two populations, to determine if one population is shifted with respect to another. The method employed is a sum of ranks comparison.

Example. To compare the difference in mean serum glucose between patients with heart failure and those without heart failure, a hypothetical study and the related measures are given below.

In patients with heart failure group, n = 25 and mean (SD) glucose = 129.2 (91.59) mg/dL.

In the comparison group (i.e., those without heart failure), n = 25 and mean (SD) glucose = 107.76 (44.41) mg dL Fig. 4.12 depicts the distribution of serum glucose levels by the two groups. It is evident from the figure that the serum glucose levels are not normally distributed by heart failure status in the study sample. Using t-test to examine their mean differences is not appropriate. In the case, we can either try to translate the data (serum glucose level) into a normally distributed (or an approximately normal) dataset, then using t-test, or we can apply Wilcoxon signed rank test to examine their mean difference.

SAS computing

SAS Proc step. The following statements request a Wilcoxon test of the null hypothesis that there is no difference in mean serum glucose (SGP) levels between the two groups. HF is the CLASS variable (represents those with or without heart failure), and SGP is the analysis variable. The WILCOXON option requests an analysis of Wilcoxon scores because the sample size

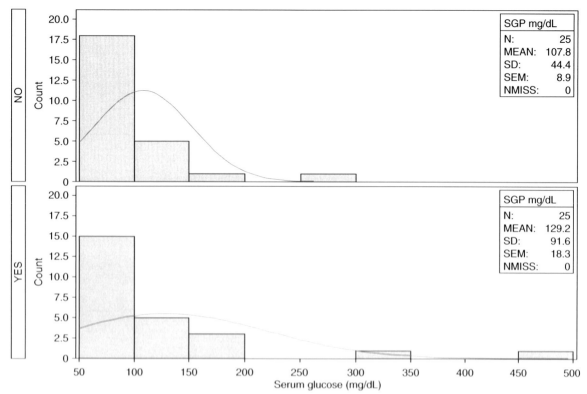

FIG. 4.12 The distribution of serum glucose (SGP, mg/dL) in patients with heart failure (n = 25) and those without heart failure (n = 25) in a hypothetical study.

is small and the large-sample normal approximation is not adequate. These statements produce the results shown below.

```
PROC NPAR1WAY WILCOXON DATA=HFBKHF25;
    CLASS HF;
        VAR SGP;
RUN;
```

Output

The NPAR1WAY Procedure

Wilcoxon Scores (Rank Sums) for Variable SGP
Classified by Variable HF

HF	N	Sum of Scores	Expected Under H0	Std Dev Under H0	Mean Score
YES	25	651.0	637.50	51.497969	26.040
NO	25	624.0	637.50	51.497969	24.960

Average scores were used for ties.

Wilcoxon Two-Sample Test

Statistic	651.0000

Normal approximation

z	0.2524
One-sided P > z	0.4004
Two-sided P > |z|	0.8007

t approximation

One-sided P > z	0.4009
Two-sided P > |z|	0.8018

z includes a continuity correction of 0.5.

Kruskal Wallis Test

Chi-square	0.0687
DF	1
P > Chi-square	0.7932

The table above displays the results of the Wilcoxon two-sample test. The Wilcoxon statistic equals 651.0.

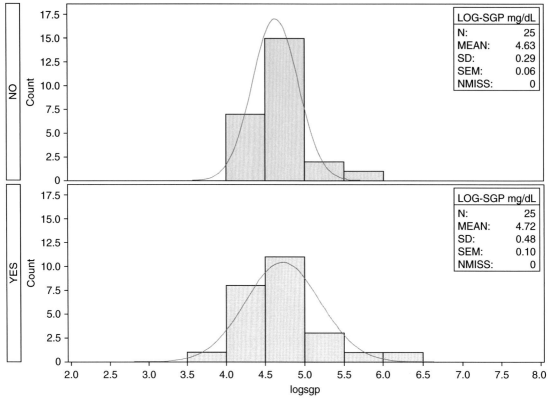

FIG. 4.13 The distribution of Log-transformed serum glucose (SGP, mg/dL) in patients with heart failure (n = 25) and those without heart failure (n = 25) in a hypothetical study.

Because this value is greater than 637.50, the expected value under the null hypothesis, PROC NPAR1WAY displays the right-sided P-values. The t approximation for the Wilcoxon scores (rank sums) two-sample test yields a two-sided P-value of 0.8018 (>.05). The result accepts the hull hypothesis that the two mean Wilcoxon scores are not statistically significant.

In practice, let us also conduct a log-transformed analysis for the purpose of using t-test. Fig. 4.13 depicts the distributions of log-transformed values of serum glucose concentration. It shows an approximately normal distribution for those with or without heart failure. Therefore, we may use t-test for the transformed data.

SAS Proc step

```
PROC TTEST DATA = HFBKHF25;
  CLASS HF;
  VAR LOGSGP;
  RUN;
```

The t-test procedure
Variable: Logsgp

HF	N	Mean	Std Dev	Std Err	Minimum	Maximum
NO	25	4.6286	0.2932	0.0586	4.2905	5.6525
YES	25	4.7219	0.4797	0.0959	3.9318	6.1717
Diff (1–2)		−0.0932	0.3976	0.1125		

HF	Method	Mean	95% CL Mean		Std Dev	95% CL Std Dev	
NO		4.6286	4.5076	4.7497	0.2932	0.2290	0.4079
YES		4.7219	4.5238	4.9199	0.4797	0.3746	0.6674
Diff (1–2)	Pooled	−0.0932	−0.3193	0.1329	0.3976	0.3315	0.4967
Diff (1–2)	Satterthwaite	−0.0932	−0.3205	0.1341			

Method	Variances	DF	t Value	P > |t|
Pooled	Equal	48	−0.83	.4112
Satterthwaite	Unequal	39.735	−0.83	**.4121**

Equality of Variances				
Method	Num DF	Den DF	F Value	P > F
Folded F	24	24	2.68	0.0192

The results from the tables above indicate the calculated t statistic = −0.83 and get a P-value of 0.4121 (for variances = unequal, because of the equality of variance test, P = .0192). The P-value of 0.4121 is >.05; therefore, we accept the null hypothesis that these two means of log values of serum glucose are not statistically significant between those with or without heart failure. The conclusion is the same as the Wilcoxon scores (rank sums) two-sample test.

The Kruskal-Wallis test mean difference among three or more than groups

The Kruskal-Wallis test, a median test, can be considered as a backup method for ANOVA where the independent variable is categorical (three or more than three groups) but the dependent variable is not normally distributed.

Example. This example is to test means difference in serum glucose levels among nonsmokers, former smokers, and current smokers. The table below shows that among nonsmokers (n = 18), mean (SD) serum glucose = 111.32 (53.44) mg/dL, in former smokers (n = 7), mean (SD) glucose = 96.29 (20.84) mg/dL, and in current smokers (n = 15), mean glucose (SD) = 142.20 (107.36) mg/dL. In biostatistics test, the null hypothesis is that these three-sample means are from the sample population, $\mu 1 = \mu 2 = \mu 3$.

The MEANS Procedure

Analysis Variable: SGP Serum Glucose (mg/dL)

SMOKING	N Obs	N	Mean	Std Dev	Minimum	Maximum
NO	28	28	111.32	53.44	73.00	334.00
FORMER	7	7	96.29	20.84	73.00	139.00
CURRENT	15	15	142.20	107.36	51.00	479.00

SAS Proc step (SMK = smoking status)

```
PROC NPAR1WAY WILCOXON DATA=HFBKHF25;
    CLASS SMK;
    VAR SGP;
    RUN;
```

The NPAR1WAY Procedure

Wilcoxon Scores (Rank Sums) for Variable SGP Classified by Variable smk

smk	N	Sum of Scores	Expected Under H0	Std Dev Under H0	Mean Score
NO	28	673.50	714.00	51.125839	24.053571
CURRENT	15	454.00	382.50	47.198668	30.266667
FORMER	7	147.50	178.50	35.738255	21.071429

Average scores were used for ties.

Kruskal-Wallis Test

Chi-square	2.5296
DF	2
P > Chi-square	.2823

In a nonparametric test for three or more than three means, we see the result of "Kruskal Wallis Test." In the example, the P value is .2823 (>.05), so we accept the null hypothesis, and there is no sufficient evidence to reject the hypothesis that the populations of serum glucose levels from the three exposures (nonsmokers, former smokers, and current smokers) have equal medians.

ANALYTICAL BIOSTATISTICS (III)
Correlation and Regression Analysis for Two Continuous Variables

Research question: In HFKBBGI dataset, we may be interested in testing whether there is a correlation between body mass index (a measure of body fat)

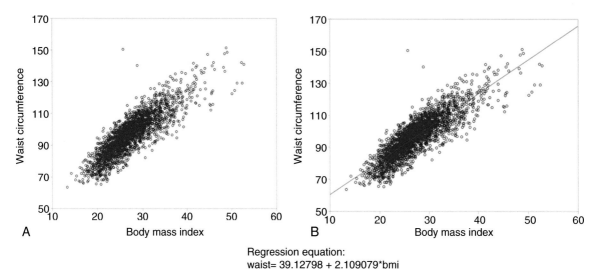

Regression equation:
waist= 39.12798 + 2.109079*bmi

FIG. 4.14 Correlation between body mass index (BMI) and waist circumference (WC) **(A)**, and linear regression model between BMI and WC **(B)**.

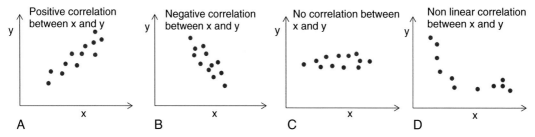

FIG. 4.15 Patterns of correlation. **(A)** Positive correlation. **(B)** Negative correlation. **(C)** No correlation. **(D)** Nonlinear correlation.

and waist (abdominal) circumference (a measure of abdominal obesity). If any, what is their quantitative relation? This research question is relevant to the method of correlation and regression analysis.

Let us start with simple linear correlation and regression analysis.

Correlation

A correlation examines the relationship between two measured variables. Linear correlation is a measure of the linear relationship between two variables measured on a numerical scale.

Linear regression

Linear regression is to model the relationship between a dependent variable (Y) and one or more independent variables (X_i).

Example. Fig. 4.14A shows the scatterplot of body mass index (BMI, kg/m^2) and waist circumference (WC in cm). It indicates that the increases in WC are associated with the increases in BMI (called a positive correlation). Fig. 4.14B depicts the linear regression line of WC with BMI (Waist = 39.13 + 2.11*BMI).

Types of correlation

There are, in general, four types of correlation: positive (linear) correlation, negative (linear) correlation, no correlation, and curve relationship (i.e., nonlinear correlation).

The following scatterplots provide a way to show a correlation between two variables graphically. Fig. 4.15 depicts four possible correlations.

How to quantify a correlation?

Correlation coefficient. To quantify whether a linear correlation exists between two variables, we calculate two types of correlation coefficients.

Pearson correlation. Pearson correlation coefficient (symbolized r) is a parametric statistic and used for data in normal or in an approximately normal distribution. The absolute value of correlation coefficient indicates the strength of the association, and the positive or negative indicates the direction of their association between two (continuous) variables.

Spearman correlation. Spearman correlation coefficient (symbolized r_s) is a nonparametric statistic and used for data that is not normally distributed or with an unknown distribution. The value of Spearman correlation coefficient indicates the direction and strength of a rank association between two variables.

Remember that a value of correlation coefficient (i.e., r or r_s) from samples is always just an estimate for an unknown population value (i.e., the population correlation coefficient, symbolized ρ—pronounced as "rho"). That, these measures from samples should be tested using an appropriate statistic method (see significant testing section).

The formula below shows the calculation of Pearson correlation coefficient (r) between two variables (such as x and y).

$$ r = \frac{\sum (x - \bar{x})(y - \bar{y})}{\sqrt{\sum (x - \bar{x})^2 \sum (y - \bar{y})^2}} $$

where x stands for the independent variable and y for the dependent variable. $\bar{X}$ is the mean value for X_1 to X_i and y is the mean value for y_1 to y_i, where $i = n$.

Properties of Pearson correlation

Pearson correlation measures the degree to which a straight line completely describes the relationship. It reaches its maximum positive or negative values when a straight line can be drawn to connect all the points in the plot. Thus (1) the correlation coefficient (r) will be 1.0 if a line could be drawn, pass through every point in the plot, and if the association is positive. This is a "perfect positive" relationship. 1.0 is the largest possible value for the correlation. Positive associations, even if the r does not equal 1, are those in which one variable increase as the other variable increases. (2) r will be −1 if a line could be drawn that would pass through every point, but the association is negative. This is a "perfect negative" relationship. −1 is the smallest possible value

for r. Negative associations are those in which one variable increases whereas the other decreases. If the estimated value of a linear correlation coefficient is closer to 1 (either +1 or −1), it indicates these two factors of interest are more strongly correlated than those with a smaller r. (3) r will be 0 when there is no straight line ascending or descending relationship.

Independent and dependent variable

From the sample of BMI and WC, we are interested in examining whether subjects who have higher BMI have higher WC. In other words, whether we could use the changes in BMI to explain the changes in WC, in the situation, we call BMI as the independent (or explanatory) variable (symbolized x) and WC is the dependent (or outcome) variable (symbolized y).

Example, using data (n = 2365) from Table 4.9 (it shows the first 10 subjects), we can calculate $\sum (x - \bar{x}) * (y - \bar{y})$, $\sum (x - \bar{x})^2$, $\sum (y - \bar{y})^2$, and then we can calculate the correlation coefficient (r):

$$ r = \frac{\sum (x - \bar{x})(y - \bar{y})}{\sqrt{\sum (x - \bar{x})^2 \sum (y - \bar{y})^2}} $$
$$ r = 0.85 $$

The estimated correlation coefficient is 0.85. Assume if we have an additional sample to examine the correlation between BMI and WC, then we would get a new correlation coefficient; these two correlation coefficients do not be exactly equal. In general, a correlation coefficient with a larger value represents a stronger correlation than those with a smaller value. The question is how large a correlation coefficient value should be? Although there is no a standard answer, Colton (1974) gave a crude rule of thumb for interpreting the size of correlation (Table 4.10).[10]

The same as the previous discussion in t test and ANOVA test, an estimated correlation coefficient (r) is a sample study. We need to test whether this statistic value is statistically significant from its population correlation coefficient (symbolized ρ).

Example. To test the correlation confident from the study of the relationship between BMI and WC, we use a t test, the formulas as below.

$$ t = \frac{r \sqrt{n - 2}}{\sqrt{1 - r^2}} $$

where r is the correlation coefficient and n is the total sample size.

TABLE 4.9
BMI and WC (Listed the First 10 Subjects)

ID	BMI (x)	WC (y)
1	37	108.5
2	25.1	91.5
3	31.1	103
4	20.4	77.7
5	24.2	102.7
6	24.2	77.9
7	23.6	88.5
8	21.1	78.3
9	25.8	89.6
10	37.6	131
Mean (n=2365)	27.44	96.99

BMI, body mass index; *WC*, waist circumference.

TABLE 4.10
Reference of the Size of a Correlation

Correlation Coefficient (r)	Interpreting
0 to 0.25 (or 0 to −0.25)	Little or no relationship
0.25 to 0.50 (or −0.25 to −0.50)	Fair degree of relationship
0.50 to 0.75 (or −0.50 to −0.75)	Moderate to good relationship
>0.70 (or <−0.75)	Very good to excellent relationship

Steps of testing a hypothesis

Step 1: Set up hypotheses:

Null hypothesis (H_0): There is no relationship between BMI and WC, i.e., $\rho = 0$.

Alternative hypothesis (H_1): $\rho \neq 0$.

Step 2: Select significance level: $\alpha = 0.01$.

Step 3: Select test statistic and calculate it.

$$t = \frac{r\sqrt{n-2}}{\sqrt{1-r^2}} = \frac{0.85\sqrt{2365-2}}{\sqrt{1-0.85^2}} = 58.03$$

Step 4: *P*-value and conclusion.

Because the sample size is big enough, t distribution is close to u distribution; we use 2.56 as the t distribution value to the corresponding *P* value of <.01.

The estimated $t = 58.03$ (>2.56). Therefore, $P < .01$, we reject the null hypothesis and accept the alternative hypothesis that these two variables are significantly correlated.

It should be noted that the significance level (i.e., α level) defines the sensitivity of the test. A value of ≤ 0.05 (or $\leq .01$) means that the error rate you are willing to accept is $\leq 5\%$ (or $\leq .01$). If we reject an "in-fact-true" H_0, we will make an error, called type I error. The choice of α ("alpha") is somewhat arbitrary, although in practice values of 0.05 and 0.01 are commonly used.

Coefficient of determination (R-square)

The coefficient of determination (denoted R^2) is another important statistic in regression analysis. It estimates the proportion of the variation in the dependent variable that is predictable from the independent variable(s).

The coefficient of determination (R^2) = correlation coefficient square.

Example. In BMI and WC, the coefficient of determination $= 0.85^2 = 0.7225$. It indicates that 72.25% of the variation in the values of WC may be accounted by the values of BMI.

Spearman correlation

In Pearson correlation analysis, the two variables of interest should be in a normal or approximately normal distribution. However, if these variables are not normally distributed, or they are ordinal or ranked variables, analysis using Pearson correlation is adequate. In the case, we should use Spearman correlation analysis, a nonparametric analysis method, which is also called rank correlation. Both Pearson and Spearman correlation coefficients can be calculated easily using computing software.

SAS computing

SAS computing is used to estimate Pearson and Spearman correlation coefficient and have significant test.

SAS Proc step

PROC CORR PEARSON SPEARMAN DATA = HFBKBG2;
VAR **BMI WAIST**;
TITLE 'Correlation analysis';
RUN;

Output: The CORR procedure

Two Variables						BMI, Waist	
Simple Statistics Variable	N	Mean	Std Dev	Median	Minimum	Maximum	Label
BMI	2642	27.34474	5.51505	26.70000	12.80000	54.30000	Body mass index
waist	2367	97.00114	13.16218	97.10000	63.50000	151.20000	Waist circumference

Pearson Correlation Coefficients $P > |r|$ under H0: Rho = 0 Number of Observations

	BMI	Waist
BMI	1.00000	0.85328
		<0.0001
Body mass index	2642	2365
waist	0.85328	1.00000
	<0.0001	
Waist circumference	2365	2367

Spearman Correlation Coefficients $P > |r|$ under H0: Rho = 0 Number of Observations

	BMI	waist
BMI	1.00000	0.85680
		<0.0001
Body mass index	2642	2365
waist	0.85680	1.00000
	<0.0001	
Waist circumference	2365	2367

Limitation of correlation coefficient
- The values of correlation coefficients (i.e., Pearson and Spearman) indicate the strength of the relationship and their direction (positive or negative) between the two variables (Fig. 4.16). It does not necessarily represent any causality.
- If the points on a curve (Fig. 4.16D) can be partially represented by a line, in this situation, the Pearson and Spearman correlations would not be zero because y does increase as x increases. The increase is simply not linear. Then a curve relationship analysis is expected.
- If the study variables of interest have extreme values (i.e., outliers), the results of correlation analysis can be dramatically affected. In the situation, evaluation for any outliers can be examined first using scatter figures, and then sensitive analysis should be carried out either excluding the outliers from the data analysis or having data transformed, such as log trans-

formation according to the nature of the dataset and purpose of the data analysis.
- A correlation may be accidental or due to a third, unmeasured factor. A careful data analysis approach should be designed and conducted.

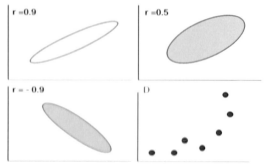

FIG. 4.16 Possible strength of the relationship between two variables.

Linear regression analysis

A correlation coefficient indicates the relationship between two variables. Our further interest may request whether we can fit a regression model (equation) to indicate the association between two factors.

We can use the formula below to fit a linear regression model. It describes the relationship between two variables (Fig. 4.17).

$$\hat{Y} = a + bx$$
$$b = \left[\sum (x - \bar{x}) * (y - \bar{y}) / \sum (x - \bar{x})^2 \right]$$
$$a = \bar{y} - b\bar{x}$$

where ŷ (Y – hat) is the predicted value of Y given a certain x, a is the intercept, and b is the regression coefficient estimated by a study sample.

Example, using the same data (n = 2365), Table 4.8 (note, this table only shows the first 10 subjects' values).

$$b = [\sum (x - \bar{x}) * (y - \bar{y})] / \sum (x - \bar{x})^2$$
$$= 2.11$$
$$a = \bar{y} - b\bar{x}$$
$$= 39.13$$
$$\text{Then, } \hat{Y} = 39.13 + 2.11x$$

In this example, WC, the dependent variable is said to be regressed on BMI, and the regression equation is written as $\hat{Y} = 39.13 + 2.11x$, where $\hat{Y}$ is the predicted WC (cm) and x is the BMI (kg/m²), the independent variable. The regression coefficient (b) > 0 indicates a positive relationship between BMI and WC.

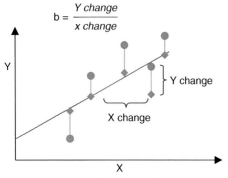

FIG. 4.17 Regression of y on x.

The regression coefficient (also called slope) of 2.11 indicates that each time a subject's BMI increases by 1 unit, his/her predicted WC increases by approximately 2.11.

As the estimated slope from a sample study, we need to test whether it is significantly from the true slope and to test whether this regression relationship of WC with BMI exists. We use the following t-test formula to test the significance of slop.

$$t = slope \div standard\ error\ of\ slope$$

$$\text{Standard error of slope} = \sqrt{s_{xy}^2 \left[\frac{1}{n} + \frac{\bar{x}^2}{\sum \left(X - \bar{X}^2\right)} \right]}$$

s_{xy} is the standard error of the estimate. It is to see the difference between the observed y and the estimated ŷ. It can be calculated using the formula below.

$$S_{xy} = \sqrt{\frac{\sum (y - \hat{y})^2}{n - 2}}$$

Example. In BMI and WC relationship study:

Step 1: H_0: the population regression coefficient = 0; alternative hypothesis, $H_1 \neq 0$

Step 2: Select significant level, $\alpha = 0.01$

Step 3: Select test statistic and calculation:

$$t = slope/standard\ error\ of\ slope$$
$$t = 2.11 \div 0.0265$$
$$= 79.62$$

Step 4: *P*-value and conclusion.

Because the sample size is big enough, t distribution is close to a normal distribution; we can use normal distribution *P*-value of 0.01 = 2.58. Our calculated t = 79.54 > 2.85, therefore, rejects the null hypothesis and accepts the alternative hypothesis. We conclude that the evidence is sufficient to show that the regression coefficient is significantly different from zero for the regression of WC on BMI.

SAS computing

SAS Proc step

```
PROC REG DATA = HFBKBG2;
MODEL WAIST = BMI;
RUN;
```

Output

Parameter Estimates

Variable	Label	DF	Parameter Estimate	Standard Error	t Value	P > |t|
Intercept	Intercept	1	39.12798	0.74106	52.80	<.0001
BMI	Body mass index	1	2.10908	0.02651	79.54	<.0001

Assumptions in regression

- For each value of the X (independent) variable, the Y (dependent) variable is assumed to have a normal distribution, and the mean of the distribution is assumed to be the predicted value $\hat{Y}$.
- No matter the value of the X variable, the SD of Y is assumed to be the same.
- The linear line assumption requires that the mean values of Y corresponding to various values of X fall in a straight line.

Association Analysis and Hypothesis Testing for Categorical Variables

Chi-square test

Research question. In Chapter 3, we discussed an example: a cross-sectional study (n = 3000) aimed to describe the frequencies of diabetes and heart failure and to examine if there was an association between diabetes and heart failure in a population aged 45 and older. Among subjects (n = 411) with diabetes mellitus (DM) the prevalence of heart failure was 16.83% (70/416), and among those without DM (n = 2584) the prevalence of heart failure was 5.53% (143/2584). The results suggest that patients with DM had a higher prevalence of heart failure than those without DM. Our further question is whether the difference in the two prevalence rates of heart failure (16.83% and 5.53%) is statistically significant. To answer this question, we apply chi-square test for 2 × 2 table to demonstrate the basics of a chi-square test.

Chi-square is a nonparametric test of statistical significance for bivariate tabular analysis. It gives an investigator the degree of confidence that whether a null hypothesis should accept or reject. Typically, the hypothesis tested with chi-square is whether two different samples (of people, such as those with or without DM) are different enough in some characteristics (such as heart failure rates). That, we can generalize from the samples that the populations from which the samples are drawn are also different in the characteristics.

The logic of the chi-square test. The total number of observations in each column (i.e., 213 and 2787) and the total number of observations in each row (i.e., 416 and 2584) (Table 4.11 on the left side) are considered to be given or fixed.

If we assume that columns and rows are independent, we can calculate the number of observations expected to occur by chance in each cell i (a, b, c, and d)—the expected frequencies.

For example, the proportion of heart failure was 16.83% in patients with DM (70/416) and 5.53% (143/2584) for those without DM. Assuming, if there was no difference regardless of the exposure to DM, the rate of heart failure in those with or without DM would be the same (i.e., 213/3000 = 7.10%) in both study samples. If this assumption was true, the expected frequency of heart failure in patients with DM (i.e., cell a) = 416 × 7.10% = 29.5 or cell a = (213 × 416)/3000 = 29.5; cell b = 416 − 29.5 = 386.5; cell c = 213 − 29.5 = 183.5; and cell d = 2584 − 183.5 = 2400.5.

If the assumption is correct, the differences between the observed frequency and the expected frequency in cells a, b, c, and d occur by chance.

The chi-square test compares the observed frequency in each cell with the expected frequency. The formula is given as follows:

$$X^2_{df} = \sum \left[\frac{(O_i - E_i)^2}{E_i} \right]$$

where O is the observed number in cell i, E is the expected number of cell i, and df stands for the degree of freedom.

$$\text{Chi-square df} = (\text{row} - 1) \times (\text{column} - 1)$$

TABLE 4.11
Observed and Expected Number of Cases in Cells a, b, c, and d

	OBSERVED				EXPECTED		
Exposure (DM)	**Heart Failure**		**Total**	**Exposure (DM)**	**Heart Failure**		**Total**
	Yes	**No**			**Positive**	**Negative**	
Yes	70 (a)	346 (b)	416	Yes	29.5 (a)	386.5 (b)	416 (a + b)
No	143 (c)	2441 (d)	2584	No	183.5 (c)	2400.5 (d)	2584 (c + d)
Total	213	2787	3000	Total	213	2787	3000
				Total	(a + c)	(b + d)	(a + b + c + d)

DM, diabetes mellitus

The chi-square formula above indicates that the values of chi-square are always positive. Fig. 4.18 depicts the distribution of chi-square at a different degree of freedom, and Table 4.12 shows the values of a chi-square statistic corresponding to the probabilities. For example, when df = 1 and $X^2 = 3.841$, the probability under the chi-square distribution is 0.05 (in red).

Significance test level in chi-square test. Table 4.12 shows part of the chi-square probabilities (df ≤ 10). In a 2×2 table, df = (row − 1) × (column − 1) = (2 − 1) × (2 − 1) = 1. Therefore,

$X^2_{df} = 1 = 3.841$ at P-value = .05, and $X^2 df = 1 = 6.635$ at P-value = .01

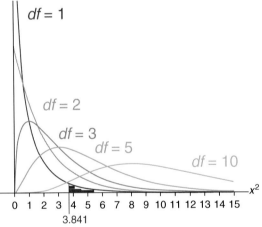

FIG. 4.18 Chi-square distribution.

Example. To test the difference in heart failure rates between individuals with or without DM:

Step 1: Hypothesis

Null hypothesis: no difference in heart failure rates between individuals with or without DM.

Alternative hypothesis: they are different.

Step 2: Select significance level: $\alpha = 0.01$

Step 3: Test statistic

$$X^2_{df} = \sum \left[\frac{(O_i - E_i)^2}{E_i} \right]$$

$$= \left[\begin{array}{l} ((70 - 29.5)^2 / 29.5) + ((346 - 386.5)^2 / 386.5) \\ + ((143 - 183.5)^2 / 183.5) \\ + ((2441 - 2400.5)^2 / 2400.5) \end{array} \right]$$

$$= 69.28$$

Step 4: P-value and conclusion

Look at chi-square table (Table 4.12), when a df = (row − 1) × (column − 1) = (2 − 1) × (2 − 1) = 1, and significance level at $P \le .01$, the chi-square statistic = 6.635. Now, the estimated $X^2_{df = 1} = 69.28$; it is larger than 6.635; therefore, the probability is <.01, reject the null hypothesis, and accept the alternative hypothesis. The differences in the prevalence of heart failure are significant between individuals with and without DM. Persons with DM had significantly higher rate than those without DM (i.e., 16.83% vs. 5.53%, $P < .01$).

SAS computing
SAS Proc step

```
PROC FREQ DATA = HFBKBG2;
TABLES DM2*HF2 /NOCOL CHISQ;
RUN;
```

TABLE 4.12
Chi-Square Probabilities

df	0.995	0.99	0.975	0.95	0.9	0.1	0.05	0.025	0.01	0.005
1	–	–	0.001	0.004	0.016	2.706	3.841	5.024	6.635	7.879
2	0.01	0.02	0.051	0.103	0.211	4.605	5.991	7.378	9.21	10.597
3	0.072	0.115	0.216	0.352	0.584	6.251	7.815	9.348	11.345	12.838
4	0.207	0.297	0.484	0.711	1.064	7.779	9.488	11.143	13.277	14.86
5	0.412	0.554	0.831	1.145	1.61	9.236	11.07	12.833	15.086	16.75
6	0.676	0.872	1.237	1.635	2.204	10.645	12.592	14.449	16.812	18.548
7	0.989	1.239	1.69	2.167	2.833	12.017	14.067	16.013	18.475	20.278
8	1.344	1.646	2.18	2.733	3.49	13.362	15.507	17.535	20.09	21.955
9	1.735	2.088	2.7	3.325	4.168	14.684	16.919	19.023	21.666	23.589
10	2.156	2.558	3.247	3.94	4.865	15.987	18.307	20.483	23.209	25.188

df, degree of freedom.

SAS Output

Statistics for Table of DM2 by HF2

Statistic	DF	Value	P
Chi-Square	1	69.2786	<.0001

Logistic regression analysis

Logistic regression analysis is applied to test a dependent variable (Y) in dichotomies (yes vs. no, positive vs. negative, died vs. alive, etc.), or in categorical, or ordinal about one or more independent variables (X_i).

Basic concept of logistic regression. The logistic regression is simply a nonlinear transformation of the linear regression. The "logistic" distribution is an S-shaped distribution function. The logit distribution contains the estimated probabilities to lie between 0 and 1. Fig. 4.19 depicts the logit distribution.

$$\text{The Logistic function } \sigma(\chi) = \frac{1}{1 + \exp(-\chi)}$$

How logistic regression works?

Logistic regression is a technique for analyzing problems in which there are one or more independent variables that determine a dependent variable (outcome). In most cases, the dependent variable is a dichotomous variable (in which there are only two possible outcomes).

The goal of logistic regression is to find the best fitting model to describe the relationship between the dichotomous characteristic of interest (dependent variable) and a set of independent (predictor or explanatory) variables. Logistic regression generates the coefficients (and its standard errors and significance levels) of a formula to predict a *logit transformation* of the probability of a presence of the characteristic of interest:

$$\text{Logit } (p) = b_0 + b_1 X_1 + b_2 X_2 + b_3 X_3 + L + b_i X_i$$

where p is the probability of the presence of the characteristic of interest and b_i is the regression coefficient for X_i.

Mathematically, logistic regression uses a maximum likelihood estimation procedure rather than the least squares estimation procedure that is used in linear regression.

The logit transformation is defined as the logged odds:

$$\text{Odds} = \frac{P}{1-P} = \frac{\text{probability presence of the characteristic}}{-\text{probability of absence of characteristic}}$$

$$\text{Logit } (P) = Ln\left[\frac{P}{1-P}\right] = b_0 + b_i X_i$$

where P is the probability that the event Y occurs, $P = (Y = 1)$; $P/(1-P)$ is the "odds ratio"; and $\ln [P/(1-P)]$ is the log odds ratio or "logit."

The equation may also be inverted to give an expression for the probability P as

$$P_X = \frac{1}{1 + \exp[-(b_0 + b_1 X_1 + b_2 X_2 + b_i X_i + b_i X_i)]}$$

Odds ratio $(OR) = \exp(b)$

Note the logistic regression formula is little complicated. However, this work of calculation can be done quickly by computer software, such as SAS.

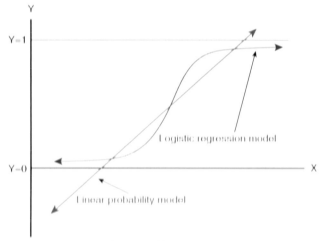

FIG. 4.19 Linear and logistic regression lines.

Interpreting logistic coefficients

Similar to what we discussed in linear regression analysis, logistic regression coefficients (b_i, sometimes called slope) can be interpreted as the effect of a unit of change in X_i variable on the predicted logits with the other variables in the model held constant. That is, how a one unit change in X_i effects the log of the odds when the other variables in the model held constant.

Interpreting odds ratios

Odds ratios in logistic regression can be interpreted as the effect of a one-unit change in X_i on the predicted odds ratio with the other variables in the model held constant.

Example. Let us use the example used in Chapter 3 again; in a cross-sectional study (n = 3000), investigators aimed to describe the frequencies of diabetes and heart failure and to examine if there was an association between diabetes and heart failure in a population aged 45 and older. Among subjects (n = 411) with DM the prevalence of heart failure was 16.83% (70/416), and among those without DM (n = 2584) the prevalence of heart failure was 5.53% (143/2584). The results suggest that patients with DM had a higher prevalence of heart failure than those without DM. Our further question is whether the difference in the two prevalence rates of heart failure (16.83% and 5.53%) is statistically significant? And what is the odds ratio of heart failure in patients with DM versus those without DM? We can apply logistic regression analysis to answer these two questions. Because the dataset has a large sample size, we apply SAS computing to estimate association and odd ratio.

SAS Proc step

```
PROC LOGISTIC DESCENDING DATA = HFBKBG2;
MODEL HF = DM /RISKLIMITS;
TITLE 'LOGISTIC REGRESSION ANALYSIS';
RUN;
```

Output

Analysis of Maximum Likelihood Estimates

Parameter	DF	Estimate	Standard Error	Wald Chi-Square	$P >$ ChiSq
Intercept	1	−2.8373	0.0860	1087.4955	<.0001
DM	1	1.2394	0.1568	62.4956	<.0001

Association of Predicted Probabilities and Observed Responses

Percent Concordant	28.8	Somers' D	0.204
Percent Discordant	8.3	Gamma	0.551
Percent Tied	62.9	Tau-a	0.027
Pairs	593,631	c	0.602

Odds Ratio Estimates and Wald Confidence Intervals

Effect	Unit	Estimate	95% Confidence Limits	
DM	1.0000	3.453	2.540	4.696

The results indicate that DM was the significantly associated risk of heart failure ($P < .0001$). The estimated logistic regression model can be written as follows:

$$\hat{Y} = -2.84 + 1.2394*DM$$

The odd ratio is indicated by Exp(b). For example, the odd ratio of DM for risk of heart failure is exp(1.2394) = 3.45, and its 95%CI is 2.54–4.70. It suggests that patients with DM have 3.45 times higher risk of heart failure than those without DM.

REFERENCES

1. Gordis L. *Epidemiology*. 5th ed. Toronto, Canada: Elsevier Canada; 2014.
2. Trapp BDaRG. *Basic & clinical biostatistics*. New York, NY 10041: McGraw-Hill Companies, Inc.; 2004.
3. Motulsky H. *Intuitive Biostatistics: A Nonmathematical Guide to Statistical Thinking*. USA: Oxford University Press; 2013.
4. SAS, Institute. *Base SAS 9.3 Procedures Guide: Statistical Procedures*; 2011. http://support.sas.com/documentation/onlinedoc/base/procstat93m1.pdf.
5. SAS. The Power to Know: Analytics Software & Solutions, 2016. https://www.sas.com/en_us/home.html.
6. Grundy SM, Brewer Jr HB, Cleeman JI, et al. Definition of metabolic syndrome: Report of the National Heart, Lung, and Blood Institute/American Heart Association conference on scientific issues related to definition. *Circulation.* 2004;109(3):433–438.
7. Levin ML. The occurrence of lung cancer in man. *Acta-Unio Int Contra Cancrum.* 1952;9(3):531–541.
8. Rothman K, Greenland D, Lash TL. Modern Epidemiology. Vol. 3. Philadelphia, PA: Wolters Kluwer: Lippincott Williams and Wilkins; 2008.
9. Szklo M, Nieto FJ. Epidemiology beyond the Basics. Vol. 2. Sudbury, MA: Jones and Bartlett; 2007.
10. Colton T. *Statistics in Medicine*. Boston, USA: Little Brown and Company; 1974.

CHAPTER 5

Advanced Biostatistics and Epidemiology Applied in Heart Failure Study

MULTIVARIATE LINEAR REGRESSION ANALYSIS AND MODELING

Multivariate analysis is an extension of bivariate (i.e., simple) regression in which two or more independent variables (X_i) are taken into consideration simultaneously to predict a value of a dependent variable (Y) for each subject.[1-5] The result of regression is an equation that represents the best prediction of a dependent variable from several continuous or dichotomous, or categorical independent variables. A general multivariate regression model can be expressed in the following form:

$$Y = \beta_0 + \beta_1 * X_1 + \beta_2 * X_2 + \beta_3 * X_3 + \beta_4 * X_2 \_ X_3 + \varepsilon$$

where Y is the dependent variable (outcome), $X_1 \ldots X_i$ are independent variables (predictors), $X_2\_X_3$ is the interaction term of X_2 and X_3, and ε is the estimated error. Because ε is unknown, we sometimes do not write it on.

Stratification Analysis for Linear Regression Models

Research question

Let us extend the example of the relationship between BMI and waist circumference (WC) that has been discussed in linear regression analysis (Chapter 4), in which the BMI-WC relationship is fitted in a linear regression model as $Y = 39.43 + 2.11 * x$. Fig. 5.1A shows the relationship between BMI and WC. We may have a further question, whether this BMI-WC relationship is different by sex. Fig. 5.1B shows the linear regression of BMI on WC by sex. It depicts that the BMI-WC relationship (indicated by the slopes of two linear lines) is stronger in males than that in females (Fig. 5.1B). It suggests that without the consideration of sex difference, we may either underestimate the BMI-WC relationship for males or overestimate that in females.

Stratification analysis

The following linear regression models (X_i represents BMI in subjects i, Y_i represents the estimated WC in

subject i) show the results for males and females separately. The regression coefficients (slopes) are statistically significant in males ($t = 70.32$, $P < .0001$) and females ($t = 64.00$, $P < .0001$). It indicates that each time a subject's BMI increases by 1 unit, about 2.40 cm increases in WC among males and about 2.03 cm in WC among females.

$$\text{In males: } \dot{Y}_i = 34.70 + 2.39770 * X_i$$
$$t = 70.32, P < .0001$$

$$\text{In females: } \dot{Y}_i = 38.16 + 2.03037 * X_i$$
$$t = 64.00, P < .0001$$

SAS computing—stratification by sex
Data step

```
/*READ SAS DATA*/

DATA HFBKBG2;

SET HFBKBG1;

RUN;
```

Proc step

```
PROC SORT DATA =HFBKBG2 ;

BY SEX;

RUN;



PROC REG DATA = HFBKBG2;

MODEL WAIST = BMI;

BY SEX;

TITLE 'REGRESSION BY SEX';

RUN;
```

Outputs
In males

			Parameter Estimates			
Variable	Label	DF	Parameter Estimate	Standard Error	t Value	P > |t|
Intercept	Intercept	1	34.70365	0.93186	37.24	<.0001
BMI	Body mass index	1	2.39770	0.03410	70.32	<.0001

In females

			Parameter Estimates			
Variable	Label	DF	Parameter Estimate	Standard Error	t Value	P > |t|
Intercept	Intercept	1	38.15852	0.90481	42.17	<.0001
BMI	Body mass index	1	2.03037	0.03172	64.00	<.0001

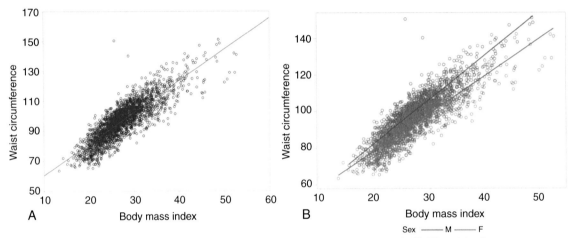

FIG. 5.1 Linear regression of body mass index (BMI) on waist circumference (WC) **(A)** and the linear regression by sex **(B)**.

Multiple Linear Regression Analysis

Multiple linear regression analysis is an extension of bivariate linear (i.e., simple) regression by having two or more independent variables.

In the example above, we have seen that sex involves in the relationship between BMI and WC. In multivariate analysis, we ask the question, "How do multiple factors interact in affecting and/or causing a relationship?" Using the same example, we apply multiple linear regression analysis methods to examine how BMI predicts changes in WC after controlling the effect of sex. The overall regression formula is shown below.

$$\hat{Y} \text{ (waist circumference)} = \beta_0 + \beta_1 * BMI + \beta_2 * Sex$$

Example, using dataset HFBKBG2 and SAS computing, sex is coded as 1 = male and 2 = female (i.e., male is the reference group for female), and the estimated regression relationship is as follows:

$$\hat{Y} \text{ (waist circumference)} = 47.53 + 2.17 * BMI \\ - 6.57 * Sex \text{ (female)}$$

The multiple regression models produce estimates of the association between BMI and WC, accounting for differences in WC due to sex. The estimated regression coefficient of BMI (2.17, t = 92.51, P < .0001) indicates that a 1-unit increase in BMI is associated with a 2.17-unit (cm) increase in WC, holding sex constant (or say, adjusted for sex). Females have lower WC, by approximately 6.57 units (coefficient = 6.7516, t = −26.37, P < .0001), holding BMI constant (or say, adjusted for BMI).

SAS computing
SAS Proc step:

PROC REG DATA = HFBKBG2;

MODEL WAIST = BMI SEX;

TITLE 'MULTIPLE LINEAR REGRESSION';

RUN;

Main output

			Parameter Estimates			
Variable	Label	DF	Parameter Estimate	Standard Error	t Value	$P > |t|$
Intercept	Intercept	1	47.53282	0.72528	65.54	<.0001
bmi	Body mass index	1	2.16541	0.02341	92.51	<.0001
sex	Sex	1	–6.57160	0.24920	–26.37	<.0001

This predicted value of WC (2.17) is different from what we got when we modeled the BMI-WC relationship separately by sex (2.40 in males and 2.03 in females). In the case, we should further test whether there is an interaction effect between sex and BMI on the changes in WC.

Interaction
By definition, an interaction is defined when a measure of a factor in the presence of two or more factors differs from the measure expected to result from their effects. The effects can be greater (positive interaction, synergism) or less (negative interaction, antagonism) than what we would expect.[6]

How to estimate and test whether an interaction effect is significant or not?
Continue using the same dataset, and we test the interaction between sex and BMI on the changes in WC. In the example, as the dependent variable is a continuous factor, we apply the analysis of covariance (ANCOVA) model to test the interaction effect.

ANCOVA
ANCOVA, an extension of analysis of variance (ANOVA), is used to test the main and interaction effects of categorical variables on a continuous dependent variable, controlling the effects of selected other variables, which covary with the dependent variable. The control variables are called the "covariates." ANCOVA does this by using statistical techniques (such as regression to partial out the effects of covariates) rather than direct experimental methods to control extraneous variables. ANCOVA is applied in experimental studies when researchers want to remove the effects of some antecedent variable. For example, pretest scores are used as covariates in pretest-posttest experimental designs. ANCOVA is also used in nonexperimental research, such as surveys or nonrandom samples, or in quasiexperiments when subjects cannot be assigned randomly to control and experimental groups. In SAS computing, we can apply Proc Reg, or Proc GLM to test an interaction effect using ANCOVA model.

Example, using dataset HFBKBG2, we add an interaction term to the multiple regression model, as shown below.

$$\acute{Y} \text{ (waist circumference)} = \beta_0 + \beta_1 * BMI + \beta_2 * Sex + \beta_3 * Sex\_BMI$$

where Sex_BMI is the interaction term of Sex and BMI.

SAS computing
Using Proc GLM to fit ANCOVA models. In the SAS Proc step below, SEX*BMI is the interaction term. The solution option is used to request that SAS print out the parameter estimates from the model.
The GLM procedure

PROC GLM DATA = HFBKBG2;

MODEL WAIST = BMI SEX SEX*BMI /SOLUTION;

RUN;

QUIT;

Main output
Dependent Variable: Waist circumference

Source	DF	Sum of Squares	Mean Square	F Value	P > F
Model	3	325,230.3093	108,410.1031	3052.48	<.0001
Error	2461	83,851.7782	35.5154		
Corrected Total	2464	409,082.0875			

	R-Square	Coeff Var	Root MSE	Waist Mean
	0.795025	6.143986	5.959477	96.99691

Source	DF	Type I SS	Mean Square	F Value	P > F
bmi	1	297,846.7100	297,846.7100	8386.42	<.0001
sex	1	25,300.7289	25,300.7289	712.39	<.0001
bmi*sex	1	2082.8705	2082.8705	58.65	<.0001

Source	DF	Type III SS	Mean Square	F Value	P > F
bmi	1	40,736.49673	40,736.49673	1147.01	<.0001
sex	1	238.85531	238.85531	6.73	.0096
bmi*sex	1	2082.87046	2082.87046	58.65	<.0001

Parameter	Estimate	Standard Error	t Value	P > |t|
Intercept	31.24878724	2.24386792	13.93	<.0001
bmi	2.76503101	0.08164250	33.87	<.0001
sex	3.45486499	1.33220720	2.59	.0096
bmi*sex	−0.36732862	0.04796581	−7.66	<.0001

We interpret the overall result by looking at the first "Source" table. We see that the model has three degrees of freedom (DF), corresponding to the three predictors included in the model (BMI, sex, and sex*BMI). The overall model is significant: F = 3052.48, $P < .0001$.

In the second table, R-square is 0.795. It indicates that 79.5% of the variation in WC could be explained by BMI, sex, and BMI_SEX interaction effect, and 20.5% is unaccounted for.

We look at the parameter estimate for the interaction effect of sex with BMI (BMI*SEX) on WC. The coefficient of interaction, β_3 (−0.3673) represents the difference in the slope of the regression line for females versus males (the reference). The estimated slope of BMI for females is about 0.37 less than for males, and this difference in slopes is significant ($t_{215} = -7.66$, $P < .0001$).

Using Proc Reg to fit ANCOVA models. SAS Data Step, we first need to create a dummy variable for categorical predictor (i.e., sex) and to create an interaction term of sex and BMI.

```
/*Multiple linear regression analysis*/

(A)   Data step, create dummy variable and interaction term;

DATA HFBKBG3;

SET HFBKBG2;

/*Create a dummy variable for female*/

if SEX =2 then SEXF =1;

else if SEX=1 then SEXF =0;   *Taking males as the reference;

/*Create interaction term OF SEXF AND BMI*/

SEXF_BMI = SEXF*BMI;

LABEL

SEXF_BMI='INTERACTION.'

;

RUN;

PROC REG DATA = HFBKBG3;

MODEL WAIST = BMI SEX SEXF_BMI /CLB;

ODS OUTPUT PARAMETERESTIMATES = PE;

RUN;
```

Outputs
The REG Procedure
Model: MODEL1
Dependent Variable: Waist circumference

Number of Observations Read	3000
Number of Observations Used	2365
Number of Observations with Missing Values	635

Analysis of Variance

Source	DF	Sum of Squares	Mean Square	F Value	P>F
Model	3	325,230	108,410	3052.48	<.0001
Error	2361	83,852	35.51537		
Corrected Total	2364	409,082			

Root MSE	5.95948	R-Square	0.7950	
Dependent Mean	96.99691	Adj R-Sq	0.7948	
Coeff Var	6.14399			

Parameter Estimates

Variable	Label	DF	Parameter Estimate	Standard Error	t Value	P>|t|	95% Confidence Limits	
Intercept	Intercept	1	31.24879	2.24387	13.93	<.0001	26.84863	35.64894
BMI	Body mass index	1	2.39770	0.03814	62.86	<.0001	2.32290	2.47250
sex	Sex	1	3.45486	1.33221	2.59	.0096	0.84245	6.06728
SEXF_BMI	INTERACTION	1	−0.36733	0.04797	−7.66	<.0001	−0.46139	−0.27327

We get the same results as we apply Proc GLM. The advantage of using Proc GLM is that we do not need to create a dummy variable and an interaction term before testing an interaction from the models.

MULTIVARIATE LOGISTIC REGRESSION ANALYSIS

Multivariate logistic regression analysis is an extension of bivariate (i.e., simple) regression in which two or more independent variables (X_i) are taken into consideration simultaneously to predict a value of a dependent variable (Y) for each subject. The dependent variable is dichotomized or categorical (i.e., multinomial or ordinal) variable when applying logistic regression models.

Example 1, using dataset HFBKBG2 to estimate risk (odds ratios) of diabetes mellitus (DM) and age for heart failure (HF). DM is coded as 1 = Yes, 0 = No; HF is coded 1 = Yes and 0 = No; and age in years. The general logistic regression model and results from SAS computing are shown below.

Logit (HF) = $\beta_0 + \beta_1 * Age + \beta_2 * DM$
Logit (HF) = $-5.37 + 0.037 * Age + 1.22 * DM$

Odds ratio = exp (β)
Odds ratio of age for HF = exp (0.037) = 1.038
Odds ratio of DM for HF = exp (1.22) = 3.387

Multivariate logistic regression analysis can be efficiently conducted using standard software, such as SAS. Tables below (SAS output) show that age (per year) and DM (yes vs. no) are significantly and positively associated with HF (yes) at P < .0001 (see table Analysis of Maximum Likelihood Estimates). The regression coefficients (standard errors) of age and DM are 0.037 (0.006) and 1.222 (0.1582), respectively. The estimate of odds ratios (OR) and 95% confidence interval (95%CI) are 10.38 (10.25–10.51) per 10 year increase in age and 3.39 (2.48–4.63) for DM (see table Odds Ratios Estimates and Wald Confidence Intervals). It suggests that individuals aged 45 and older on an average of each 10 year increase in age have 10.38 times higher risk (or on an average of 1 year increase in age has 1.038 times higher risk) of heart failure than those who are 10 years young. This association is independent of DM (i.e., holding DM constant). Patients with DM have 3.39 times higher risk of heart failure than those without DM (OR = 3.39, 95%CI: 2.49–4.63), holding age constant.

SAS computing

SAS Proc step:
Option "RISKLIMITS" requests outputs with OR and 95%CI.

PROC LOGISTIC DESCENDING DATA = HFBKBG2;

MODEL HF = AGE DM /RISKLIMITS ;

TITLE 'LOGISTIC REGRESSION ANALYSIS';

RUN;

Main output

Analysis of Maximum Likelihood Estimates

Parameter	DF	Estimate	Standard Error	Wald Chi-Square	$P > ChiSq$
Intercept	1	−5.3676	0.4512	141.5144	<.0001
age	1	0.0370	0.00625	35.0730	<.0001
DM	1	1.2215	0.1582	59.5889	<.0001

Association of Predicted Probabilities and Observed Responses

Percent Concordant	68.5	Somers' D	0.383
Percent Discordant	30.1	Gamma	0.389
Percent Tied	1.4	Tau-a	0.051
Pairs	593,631	c	0.692

Odds Ratio Estimates and Wald Confidence Intervals

Effect	Unit	Estimate	95% Confidence Limits	
age	1.0000	1.038	1.025	1.051
DM	1.0000	3.392	2.488	4.626

Interaction effect in logistic regression

The same as we discussed in multiple linear regression models, potential interaction of the predictors should be considered and tested. The formula below shows the relationship.

$$\text{Logit (HF)} = \beta_0 + \beta_1 * \text{Age} + \beta_2 * \text{DM} + \text{Age}\_\text{DM}$$

SAS computing

SAS Proc step

In SAS Proc logistic regression model, we can add the interaction term directly to the model (i.e., as shown "AGE*DM" in the model below). Meanwhile, because the model contains age as a continuous variable the ORs for AGE, DM, and AGE*DM are not shown, but the regression coefficients do. (see main output table).

PROC LOGISTIC DESCENDING DATA = HFBKBG2;

MODEL HF = AGE DM AGE*DM /RISKLIMITS;

TITLE 'LOGISTIC REGRESSION ANALYSIS';

RUN;

As the output table given below shows that the interaction effect of age and DM (coded as Age*DM) on the risk of heart failure is not statistically significant (the coefficient estimate of age*BMI is −0.0155, $P = .2884$).

Main output

Analysis of Maximum Likelihood Estimates

Parameter	DF	Estimate	Standard Error	Wald Chi-Square	$P > ChiSq$
Intercept	1	−5.6278	0.5198	117.2203	<.0001
Age	1	0.0407	0.00719	32.0377	<.0001
DM	1	2.3103	1.0341	4.9907	.0255
Age*DM	1	−0.0155	0.0146	1.1270	.2884

Association of Predicted Probabilities and Observed Responses

Percent Concordant	68.3	Somers' D	0.380
Percent Discordant	30.3	Gamma	0.386
Percent Tied	1.4	Tau-a	0.050
Pairs	593,631	C	0.690

Example 2, using data HFBKBG2 to estimate risk (odds ratios) of diabetes mellitus (DM), age, and smoking status (SMK) for heart failure (HF), DM is coded as 1 = Yes, 0 = No; HF is coded as 1 = Yes, and 0 = No; age in years; and cigarette smoking status, 0 = NO smoking, 1 = FORMER smoked, and 2 = CURRENT smoking. The general logistic regression model and results from SAS computing are shown below.

$$\text{Logit (HF)} = \beta_0 + \beta_1 * \text{Age} + \beta_2 * \text{DM} + \beta_3 * \text{SMK}$$

In Example 2, we have three predictors (independent variables): age, DM, and SMK. In the first computing model, we include these three factors in SAS Proc step. In the statement, CLASS is used for categorical variables (such as SMK). In the example, SMK has three levels (no, former, and current), we need to indicate which level is the reference group. We can indicate it as "Ref = NO." "PARAM = REF" means the relevant tests using REF as the reference group. "EXPB" has the same function as "RISKLIMITS" for computing OR.

SAS computing
SAS Proc statement

PROC LOGISTIC DESCENDING DATA = HFBKBG2;

CLASS SMK (REF='NO') / PARAM = REF;

MODEL HF = AGE DM SMK /EXPB;

TITLE 'LOGISTIC REGRESSION ANALYSIS';

RUN;

Main output

The results indicate that age, DM, and former smoked status are significantly associated with the odds of heart failure at a level of $P<.05$. The estimated OR (95%CI) of age, DM, and former smokers are 1.04 (1.03–1.05, $P<.0001$), 3.39 (2.47–4.62, $P<.0001$), and 2.13(1.42–3.19, $P=.0002$), respectively. Current smoking status is positively, but not significantly, associated with the risk of heart failure in the study sample. It should be noted that this computing is a cross-sectional analysis using the baseline survey dataset. It is very likely for some smokers who had heart failure diagnosed first and then quitted smoking because of the disease, and they became former smokers. It, at least, partially explains why we commonly see a larger OR in former smokers compared with current smokers in a cross-sectional analysis. The results suggest that individuals who are 1-year older is associated with 1.039 times higher risk of heart failure than those who are 1-year younger, holding the effects of DM and smoking status constant (or say, adjusted for DM and smoking status). Patients with DM have 3.385 times higher risk of heart failure than those without DM, holding age and smoking status constant. Former smokers have 2.131 times higher risk of heart failure than those who never smoked, holding age and DM status constant.

Analysis of Maximum Likelihood Estimates

Parameter		DF	Estimate	Standard Error	Wald Chi-Square	$P>$ChiSq	Exp(Est)
Intercept		1	−5.5890	0.4783	136.5463	<.0001	0.004
age		1	0.0383	0.00644	35.3380	<.0001	1.039
DM		1	1.2193	0.1590	58.7718	<.0001	3.385
SMK	CURRENT	1	0.1659	0.1810	0.8403	.3593	1.180
SMK	FORMER	1	0.7565	0.2057	13.5224	.0002	2.131

Odds Ratio Estimates

Effect	Point Estimate	95% Wald Confidence Limits	
Age	1.039	1.026	1.052
DM	3.385	2.478	4.623
SMK CURRENT vs NO	1.180	0.828	1.683
SMK FORMER vs NO	2.131	1.424	3.189

Association of Predicted Probabilities and Observed Responses

Percent Concordant	70.8	Somers' D	0.423
Percent Discordant	28.5	Gamma	0.426
Percent Tied	0.6	Tau-a	0.056
Pairs	593,631	C	0.711

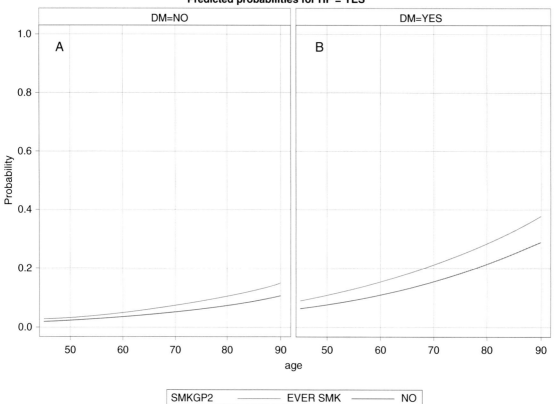

Predicted probabilities for HF = YES

FIG. 5.2 Predicated probabilities of suffering from heart failure (HF) in individuals with diabetes mellitus (DM) **(A)** and without DM **(B)** by age and smoking status.

Example 3, using SAS "Ods graphics on" statement, we can further visualize the effects of predictors on an outcome. In the example, using the same dataset HFBKBG2, SMKGP2 is coded as 1 = ever smoked (i.e., either current smoking or former smoking status) and 0 = never smoked.

The results show that age, DM, and smoking status are significantly associated with the risk of heart failure. Their estimated OR (95%CI) for heart failure are 1.04 (1.03–1.05, $P < .0001$), 3.44 (2.52–4.69, $P < .0001$), and 1.47 (1.09–1.97, $P = .0115$), respectively.

Fig. 5.2 depicts the predicted probabilities for heart failure. It shows that individuals with an increase in age are associated with the increase in the probabilities for heart failure, regardless of their DM and/or smoking status.

However, individuals with DM have higher probabilities for heart failure (Fig. 5.2B) and those who smoked (either current or former) have higher probabilities for heart failure compared with their corresponding counterparts. Most importantly, Fig. 5.2 depicts a strong jointed effect of DM and smoking on the risk of heart failure across the ages. For example, among individuals at age 80 and who have DM and who smoked, the predicted probability of heart failure is about 30%, and for those with DM, but without smoking, it is about 20% (Fig. 5.2B). However, these associations would dramatically reduce if individuals without DM and who never smoked, the probabilities for heart failure is much less than 10% at the same age or slightly above 10% in those who ever smoked (Fig 5.2A).

SAS computing
SAS Proc Statement

```
ODS GRAPHICS ON;

PROC LOGISTIC DESCENDING DATA=HFBKBG2

PLOTS(ONLY)=(ODDSRATIO(RANGE=CLIP));

    CLASS SMKGP2 (REF='NO') DM (REF='NO') /PARAM=REF;

    MODEL HF = AGE DM SMKGP2;


    ODDSRATIO SMKGP2;

    ODDSRATIO DM;

    ODDSRATIO AGE;

    CONTRAST 'PAIRWISE FORMER VS NO' SMKGP2 1 0 / ESTIMATE=EXP;

    CONTRAST 'YES VS NO' DM 0 / ESTIMATE=EXP;

    EFFECTPLOT / AT(DM=ALL) NOOBS;

    EFFECTPLOT SLICEFIT(SLICEBY=SMKGP2 PLOTBY=DM) / NOOBS;

RUN;

ODS GRAPHICS OFF;
```

Main output

Analysis of Maximum Likelihood Estimates

Parameter		DF	Estimate	Standard Error	Wald Chi-Square	$P>$ChiSq
Intercept		1	−5.6988	0.4768	142.8770	<.0001
age		1	0.0397	0.00640	38.4697	<.0001
DM	YES	1	1.2348	0.1587	60.5620	<.0001
SMKGP2	EVER SMK	1	0.3822	0.1513	6.3821	.0115

Odds Ratio Estimates

Effect	Point Estimate	95% Wald Confidence Limits	
age	1.041	1.028	1.054
DM YES vs NO	3.438	2.519	4.692
SMKGP2 EVER SMK vs NO	1.466	1.089	1.972

SURVIVAL ANALYSIS

In medical research including heart failure epidemiologic study, a prospective cohort study or a randomized clinical trial is commonly conducted to determine whether a new treatment or a new surgical procedure or a specific risk factor of interest has a significant impact on the risk of disease (incidence, severity, and/or mortality) in a given a period of follow-up. Although measures of short-term effects are of interest with efforts to provide a better-qualified healthcare, long-term outcomes, including incidence and mortality, are also important. In the study design, we examine a time-to-event association, called as survival analysis or survival modeling. Most frequently used survival analysis methods are Kaplan-Meier estimator and Cox proportional hazards regression models.

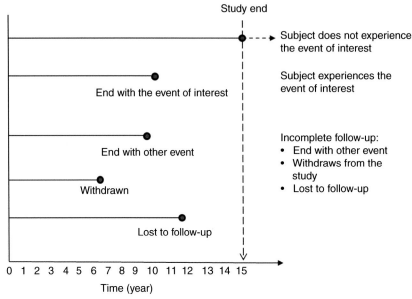

FIG. 5.3 Types of survival data.

Basic Characteristics of Survival Analysis
- Time to event
- Account for censored data
- An outcome with binary classification (i.e., an event either occurs or does not)
- Able to compare survival function between two or more groups

Time: It can be days, weeks, months, or years from the beginning of follow-up of an individual until an event occurs or at the end of follow-up.

Event: It can be incidence of disease, readmission, mortality, or becoming a different stage of disease (such as from heart failure stages A to C or D), or change to a different treatment approach (such as heart transplantation), any designed event of a study. Fig. 5.3 depicts the types of survival data.

Censoring: We do not know the time exactly (i.e., the exact survival or experienced time of an event). Specifically, in most observational prospective studies, a censoring occurs although we know an individual's follow-up time, we are not aware of the survival time exactly. It can happen that an individual does not experience the event of interest at the end of follow-up, or an individual who is lost to follow up during the study period, or an individual has to stop or withdraw from the study (such as due to an adverse drug reaction or other competing events).

Although censoring is a problem in survival analysis, to estimate the survival probability at a given time,

we make use of the risk set at that point to include the information we have on a censored individual up to the date of censorship, rather than simply throwing away all the information on a censored individual.[7] Theoretically, when time (T) goes from 0 up to infinity, the survivor function is graphed as a decreasing smooth curve, which begins at S(t) = 1 at t = 0, and S(t) monotonically decreases to zero as t increases toward infinity (Fig. 5.4A). Using data from a real setting, however, what we observed is survival curves are not smooth curves because of the data from sampling studies, which have sampling errors, censored data, and unmeasured errors. Fig. 5.4B takes the sample dataset, HFBKBGYR, as an example to depict the survival function (probability) of participants with heart failure (blue line) and those without heart failure (black line) from all-cause mortality at the end of follow-up. Similar to what have discussed in linear and logistic regression models, in survival analysis we wanted to examine a survivorship of interest between time and event from samples to draw implications about the actual survival time.

Person-year and per person-year rates
In Chapter 3, we discussed that studies with a prospective cohort design should estimate their person-years (months or days), which represents the time of an individual who has been exposed or at risk of a particular condition of interest (such as incidence and mortality). We demonstrated how to calculate person-year when

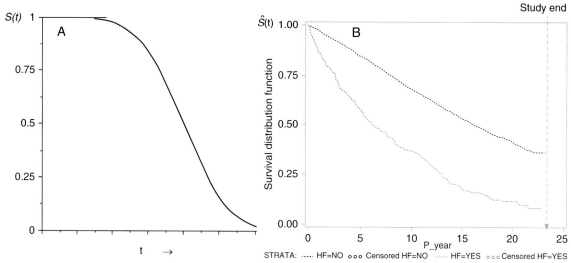

FIG. 5.4 Theoretical survival function (**A**) and example of an observed survival function (**B**).

a study with a sample size. Data from the real health-care settings, however, are much larger. It is impossible to calculate person-year rate manually. Fortunately, to date, almost all biostatistics software can do the work in few seconds when a dataset is ready.

Strategy for survival data analysis and presentation
Descriptive analysis and presentation
- Incidence and/or mortality rates per person-years
- Address key factors of interest

Survival models
- Kaplan-Meier curves
- Cox proportional hazards regression analysis

Example—rates per person-years
As we discussed before, a person-year represents the duration (e.g., year) of an individual who has exposure to a risk factor of interest.

We use data HFBKBG2YR (HFBKBG follow-up dataset) to calculate and compare all-cause mortality (per person-years) in individuals with heart failure versus those without heart failure. In HFBKBGYR, participants have a mean (median) follow-up of 13.4 (15.2) years by the end of the study. The events of interest are all-cause mortality and cardiovascular disease–specific mortality. The *International Classification of Disease, Tenth Revision* (*ICD-10*) is used to code the cause of death. All-cause mortality (death) is coded as 0 = alive and 1 = dead, and mortality from cardiovascular disease (D_CVD) is coded as 1 = dead, 0 = alive, whichever occurred first within the period of follow-up.

Research questions: What were the all-cause mortality rates per 100 person-years in individuals with heart failure and those without heart failure during the time of follow-up? What were the impacts of diabetes mellitus on all-cause mortality by heart failure status at baseline?

To answer the research questions, we apply SAS Proc GENMOD. The SAS statements and main outputs are shown below.

SAS computing
SAS Data Step: First, we need to get log-transformed values of the period of follow-up (years) for calculating mortality rates per person-years using SAS Proc GENMOD.

SAS statements and outputs:

/*log-transformation of person-year (P-Year)*/

```
DATA HFBKBG2PY;

SET HFBKBG2;

LG_PY = LOG (P_YEAR);

RUN;
```

SAS Proc step is used to calculate mortality per person-years using the SAS statement below. It should be noted that the original follow-up time (years in the case) should be log transformed (e.g., LG_PY), then be assigned to "OFFSET = LG_PY" in SAS Proc GENMOD statement. See the example below.

PROC GENMOD DATA = HFBKBG2PY;

MODEL **DEATH** = HF / DIST = POISSON OFFSET = LG_PY;

ESTIMATE "RATE FOR HF (HF=1)" **INTERCEPT** 1 **HF** 1;

ESTIMATE "RATE FOR HF (HF=0)" **INTERCEPT** 1;

ESTIMATE "RATE RATIO FOR HF(YES)/HF(NO)" **HF** 1;

RUN;

Outcome: All-cause mortality (Death: 1 = dead, 0 = alive)
Predictor: Heart Failure (HF: 1 = yes, 0 = No)

Main output

Analysis of Maximum Likelihood Parameter Estimates

Parameter	DF	Estimate	Standard Error	Wald 95% Confidence Limits		Wald Chi-Square	P > ChiSq
Intercept	1	−3.1567	0.0246	−3.2050	−3.1084	16,411.6	<.0001
HF	1	0.9435	0.0766	0.7934	1.0937	151.65	<.0001
Scale	0	1.0000	0.0000	1.0000	1.0000		

Contrast Estimate Results

Label	Mean Estimate	Mean Confidence Limits		L'Beta Estimate	Standard Error	Alpha	L'Beta Confidence Limits		Chi-Square	P > ChiSq
Rate for HF (HF = 1)	0.1094	0.0949	0.1261	−2.2131	0.0725	0.05	−2.3553	−2.0709	930.61	<.0001
Rate for HF (HF = 0)	0.0426	0.0406	0.0447	−3.1567	0.0246	0.05	−3.2050	−3.1084	16,412	<.0001
Rate ratio for HF(YES)/ HF(NO)	2.5690	2.2108	2.9853	0.9435	0.0766	0.05	0.7934	1.0937	151.65	<.0001

Results: Within a mean follow-up of 13.3 years in individuals aged 45 and older, all-cause mortality rate (95%CI) in patients with heart failure is 10.94% (9.49%–12.61%) per 100 person-years and 4.26% (4.06%–4.47%) per 100 person-years in those without heart failure. Individuals with heart failure have significantly higher all-cause mortality than those without the disease (10.94% vs. 4.26%, Chi-Square = 151.65, P<.0001).

All-cause mortality rates by DM status in individuals with or without heart failure are shown below.

SAS computing
SAS Proc statements:

PROC SORT DATA = HFBKBG2PY;

BY **DM**;

RUN;

PROC GENMOD DATA = HFBKBG2PY;

MODEL **DEATH** = HF / DIST = POISSON OFFSET = LG_PY;

ESTIMATE "RATE FOR HF (HF=1)" **INTERCEPT** 1 **HF** 1;

ESTIMATE "RATE FOR HF (HF=0)" **INTERCEPT** 1;

ESTIMATE "RATE RATIO FOR HF(YES)/HF(NO)" **HF** 1;

BY **DM**;

RUN;

Output in individuals without DM

Contrast Estimate Results

Label	Mean Estimate	Mean Confidence Limits		L'Beta Estimate	Standard Error	Alpha	L'Beta Confidence Limits		Chi-Square	P > ChiSq
Rate for HF (HF = 1)	0.0959	0.0804	0.1144	−2.3444	0.0898	0.05	−2.5204	−2.1684	681.52	<.0001
Rate for HF (HF = 0)	0.0395	0.0375	0.0417	−3.2308	0.0270	0.05	−3.2836	−3.1780	14,363	<.0001
Rate ratio for HF(YES)/ HF(NO)	2.4265	2.0191	2.9160	0.8864	0.0938	0.05	0.7027	1.0702	89.38	<.0001

Output in individuals with DM

Contrast Estimate Results

Label	Mean Estimate	Mean Confidence Limits		L'Beta Estimate	Standard Error	Alpha	L'Beta Confidence Limits		Chi-Square	P > ChiSq
Rate for HF (HF = 1)	0.1485	0.1167	0.1890	−1.9073	0.1231	0.05	−2.1486	−1.6660	240.09	<.0001
Rate for HF (HF = 0)	0.0699	0.0620	0.0787	−2.6611	0.0607	0.05	−2.7801	−2.5420	1919.0	<.0001
Rate ratio for HF(YES)/ HF(NO)	2.1250	1.6237	2.7810	0.7538	0.1373	0.05	0.4847	1.0228	30.15	<.0001

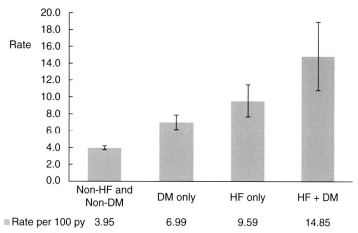

	Non-HF and Non-DM	DM only	HF only	HF + DM
Rate per 100 py	3.95	6.99	9.59	14.85

FIG. 5.5 All-cause mortality rates (per person-years [py]) by heart failure (HF) and diabetes mellitus (DM) status.All-cause mortality rate (per 100 person-years) in individuals aged ≥45 by heart failure and/or with diabetes status over a mean follow-up of 13.4 years

The results indicate that heart failure patients with comorbid DM have the highest all-cause mortality rate (14.85%, 95%CI: 11.67%–18.90%). It is then followed by those with heart failure only (9.59, 8.04%–11.44%), those with DM only (6.99, 6.20%–7.87%), and those without both heart failure and DM (3.95%, 3.75%–4.14%). In the SAS Proc statement, we may further estimate all-cause mortality rate in individuals with and without heart failure by diabetes status using frequency. The figure above depicts that people with both heart failure and DM had the highest all-cause mortality (14.85 per 100 person-years). Fig. 5.5 shows the all-cause mortality rates per 100 person-years by heart failure and comorbid DM status.

Kaplan-Meier Survival Curves and the Log-Rank Test

Kaplan-Meier survival curves and modeling (also called Kaplan-Meier estimator or the product limit estimator) is a nonparametric statistic. It involves the calculation of the probability of each event at the time it occurs. The denominator for this calculation is the population at risk at the time of each event's occurrence.[8] The Kaplan-Meier estimator was named after Edward L. Kaplan and Pau Meier, who submitted similar manuscripts individually to the *Journal of the American Statistical Association*. The journal editor, John Tukey, convinced them to combine their work into one paper, which was then published in 1958.[9]

The Kaplan-Meier estimator is a statistic; its mathematical formula can be written as follows:

$$\hat{V}ar\left(\hat{S}(t)^2\right) = \hat{S}(t)^2 \sum_{i:t_i \leq t} \frac{d_i}{n_i(n_i - d_i)},$$

where $\hat{S}(t)$ is the estimated survival function, d_i is the number of cases, and n_i is the total number of observations, for $t_i < t$.

Kaplan-Meier estimator is a univariate analysis. It estimates the survivor functions and compares survival curves between groups of individuals with the different disease and/or exposure status. Log-trend test approach is commonly used to compare survival curves by groups.

Example: using HFBKB2GPY follow-up data

Research questions: What were the survival trends in subjects with or without heart failure, and among them with or without comorbidity of diabetes? Whether were these trends statistically significant? What were the 5-year survival rates by disease status?

Using SAS, we can apply Kaplan-Meier plot to display survival curves, the number of subjects at risk, confidence limits, log-trend test, and homogeneity test *P*-value.

In the following statements, PROC LIFETEST is invoked to compute the product-limit estimate of the survivor function for each risk category. Using ODS graphics, you can display the number of subjects at risk in the survival plot. The PLOTS = option requests that the survival curves be plotted, and the ATRISK = suboption specifies the time points at which the at-risk numbers are displayed. P_YEAR is the follow-up time (years), and DEATH is the all-cause mortality (coded 1 for dead and 0 for alive). "TIMELIST=5" means for calculating 5-year survival rates. In the STRATA statement, the ADJUST = SIDAK option requests the Sidák multiple-comparison adjustment, and by default, all paired comparisons are carried out.

SAS computing

SAS Proc Step:

```
ODS GRAPHICS ON;

PROC LIFETEST DATA = HFBKBG2PY CONFTYPE=LINEAR PLOTS=SURVIVAL

(ATRISK=0 TO 23 BY 2.5) TIMELIST=5 MAXTIME=23;

TIME P_YEAR*DEATH(0);

STRATA HF DM / ORDER=INTERNAL TREND TEST = (LOGRANK) ADJUST = SIDAK;

RUN;

ODS GRAPHICS OFF;
```

Fig. 5.6 depicts four survival curves for individuals without heart failure and diabetes (blue line), individuals with diabetes only (red line), individuals with heart failure only (green line), and individuals with both heart failure and diabetes (black line). It indicates that individuals with heart failure and comorbid diabetes had the poorest survival trend among the other three groups. Test for trends are significant at $P < .001$ for those without heart failure and without DM compared with the rest of three groups. It appears that the impact of heart failure (red line) or diabetes (green line) alone on the survival curves is different, but their trends are not statistically significant ($P > .05$) compared with each other (Fig. 5.6). In the study, the 5-year survival rates are 85.52%, 77.75%, 63.64%, and 45.71% for those without heart failure and diabetes (green), followed by those with diabetes only, those with heart failure only, and those with both heart failure and diabetes, respectively.

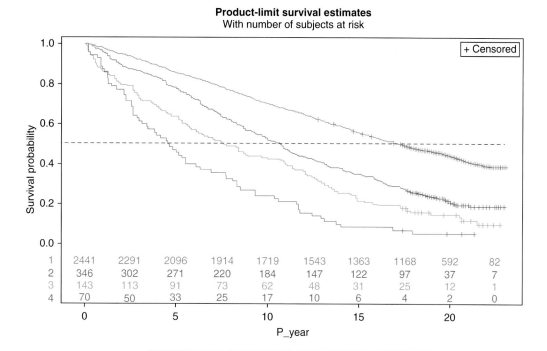

FIG. 5.6 Kaplan-Meier survival curves by heart failure (HF) and diabetes mellitus (DM) status.

Adjustment for Multiple Comparisons for the Logrank Test

| | | | P-Values | |
Stratum	_Stratum_	Chi-Square	Raw	Sidak
1	2	147.1	<.0001	<.0001
1	3	216.8	<.0001	<.0001
1	4	260.0	<.0001	<.0001
2	3	4.4820	.0343	.1887
2	4	14.8789	.0001	.0007
3	4	5.3250	0.0210	0.1197

SAS Proc statement for 5-year survival rates by heart failure and DM status is given as follows. In the SAS codes, "TIMELIST = 5" means to request for 5-year survival rates. "STRATA HF DM" means to request a stratified analysis for HF (heart failure) and DM (diabetes mellitus).

```
PROC LIFETEST DATA = HFBKBG2PY TIMELIST=5 MAXTIME=25;

TIME P_YEAR*DEATH(0);

STRATA HF DM /TREND TEST = (LOGRANKWILCOXON);

RUN;
```

Stratum 1: HF = NO, DM = NO

Product-Limit Survival Estimates

Timelist	P_year	Survival	Failure	Survival Standard Error	Number Failed	Number Left
5.00000	5.0000	0.8562	0.1438	0.00710	351	2090

Stratum 2: HF = NO, DM = YES

Product-Limit Survival Estimates

Timelist	P_year	Survival	Failure	Survival Standard Error	Number Failed	Number Left
5.00000	5.0000	0.7775	0.2225	0.0224	77	269

Stratum 3: HF = YES, DM = NO

Product-Limit Survival Estimates

Timelist	P_year	Survival	Failure	Survival Standard Error	Number Failed	Number Left
5.00000	4.7500	0.6364	0.3636	0.0402	52	91

Stratum 4: HF = YES, DM = YES

Product-Limit Survival Estimates

Timelist	P_year	Survival	Failure	Survival Standard Error	Number Failed	Number Left
5.00000	5.0000	0.4571	0.5429	0.0595	38	32

The Kaplan-Meier estimator is one of the most commonly used methods to illustrate survival curves. The disadvantage of Kaplan-Meier estimator is that it does not account for confounding or effect modification by other covariates. However, Cox proportional hazard regression models can be applied in either a univariate or a multivariate analysis (i.e., adjusting confounding effects).

Cox Proportional Hazards Regression Models

Cox proportional hazards model assumes that the underlying hazard *rate* (rather than survival time) is a function of the independent variables (and covariates). The model is expressed as follows:

$$\log\,[h(ti)/h_0(ti)] = \beta_1 X_1 + \beta_2 X_2 + \beta_3 X_3 + \cdots \beta_k X_k$$

where h(ti) is called the hazard function, i.e., the probability of having the event of interest at time ti given the subject survived at and beyond the time ti. The term $h_0(ti)$ is called the *baseline hazard*; it is the hazard for the respective individual when all independent variable values are equal to zero. Terms X_2, X_3, … X_k are covariates and β_1, β_2, … β_k are the corresponding regression coefficients.

Assumptions of Cox proportional hazards model

In Cox proportional hazards model, one of the important issues is the assumption of proportional hazards. In a regression type setting, this means that the survival curves for two or more strata (determined by the particular choices of values for the study of interest) must have hazard functions that are proportional over time (i.e., constant relative hazard).

Example: using HFBKB2GPY follow-up data

Research questions: (1) what is the hazard ratio (HR) of heart failure for the risk of all-cause mortality? (2) What are age and sex-adjusted HRs (95%CI) of heart failure for the risk of all-cause mortality? (3) What are the joint-effects of heart failure with DM on the risk of all-cause mortality?

SAS computing

In SAS Proc Step:

PROC PHREG MODEL fits the Cox model by maximizing the partial likelihood and computes the baseline survivor function by using the Breslow (1972) estimate.[7]

In the PROC PHREG MODEL statement, the response variable, P_YEAR, is crossed with the censoring variable, status (DEATH), with the value that indicates censoring is enclosed in parentheses. The values of P_YEAR are considered censored if the value of status (Death) is 0; otherwise, they are considered event times. The output statement above makes a new dataset that contains the Schoenfeld residuals.[10] One assessment of proportional hazards is based on these residuals, which ought to show no association with time if proportionality holds.

```
PROC PHREG DATA = HFBKBG2PY ;

    MODEL P_YEAR*DEATH(0)= HF / RISKLIMITS;

    OUTPUT OUT = PROPCHECK RESSCH = SCHRES;

RUN;
```

The result shows that the HR (95%CI) of heart failure for risk of all-cause mortality is 2.72 (2.34–3.16).

Main output

Analysis of Maximum Likelihood Estimates

Parameter	DF	Parameter Estimate	Standard Error	Chi-Square	$P > $ChiSq	Hazard Ratio	95% Hazard Ratio Confidence Limits	
HF	1	1.00015	0.07705	168.5039	<.0001	2.719	2.338	3.162

Fitting survivor function
By using ODS Graphics, PROC PHREG allows us to plot the survival curve for HF = 0 and the survival curve for HF = 1, but first, we must save these two covariate values in an SAS dataset as in the following DATA Step and then SAS Proc Step (Fig. 5.7).

```
DATA REGIMES;

    HF=0;

    OUTPUT;

    HF=1;

    OUTPUT;

RUN;


ODS GRAPHICS ON;

PROC PHREG DATA=HFBKBG2PY PLOT(OVERLAY)=SURVIVAL;

MODEL P_YEAR*DEATH(0)= HF;

BASELINE COVARIATES=REGIMES OUT=_NULL_;

RUN;

ODS GRAPHICS OFF;
```

Fig. 5.7 depicts that patients with heart failure had a poorer survival curve (red lime) than those without heart failure (blue line).

Age and sex-adjusted hazard ratios (95% confidence interval)
The following SAS statement aims to estimate HR of heart failure on the risk of all-cause mortality, with adjustment for age and sex.

SAS Proc Step

```
PROC PHREG DATA = HFBKBG2PY;

CLASS AGEGP4 (REF=FIRST) SEX (REF=FIRST) / PARAM =REF;

MODEL P_YEAR*DEATH(0)= AGEGP4 SEX HF /  RISKLIMITS;

RUN;
```

Main output

Analysis of Maximum Likelihood Estimates

Parameter		DF	Parameter Estimate	Standard Error	Chi-Square	P > ChiSq	Hazard Ratio	95% Hazard Ratio Confidence Limits		Label
agegp4	55–64	1	0.91846	0.10086	82.9169	<.0001	2.505	2.056	3.053	agegp4 55-64
agegp4	65–74	1	1.74186	0.09573	331.0751	<.0001	5.708	4.731	6.886	agegp4 65-74
agegp4	>=75	1	2.69803	0.09562	796.2173	<.0001	14.850	12.313	17.911	agegp4 >=75
sex	F	1	−0.29536	0.04708	39.3617	<.0001	0.744	0.679	0.816	Sex F
HF		1	0.68525	0.07741	78.3563	<.0001	1.984	1.705	2.309	

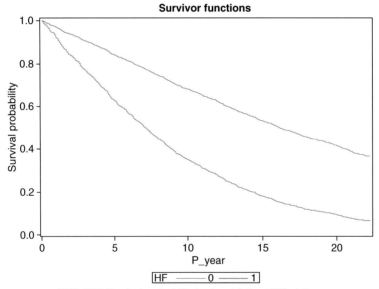

FIG. 5.7 Survival probability by heart failure (HF) status.

The table above indicates that the HR (95%CI) of heart failure for the risk of all-cause mortality was 1.984 (1.705–2.309), and this association was independent of age and sex.

Joint effects of heart failure with DM on the risk of all-cause mortality
In the joint-effect analysis, we define a 4-level exposure to heart failure and/or diabetes status.

HFDM = 0 for those without heart failure and diabetes
HFDM = 1 for those with diabetes, but without heart failure
HFDM = 2 for those with heart failure, but without diabetes
HFDM = 3 for those with heart failure and diabetes

SAS computing

```
                          /*CREATE A FOUR LEVELS DATASET*/

              DATA REG_HFDM;

                  HFDM=0;

                          OUTPUT;

                  HFDM=1;

                          OUTPUT;

                      HFDM=2;

                      OUTPUT;

                      HFDM=3;

                      OUTPUT;

              RUN;



                  /*FIT 4 LEVELS */



              ODS GRAPHICS ON;

                  PROC PHREG DATA=HFBKBG2PY PLOT(OVERLAY)=SURVIVAL;

                  CLASS  HFDM (REF=FIRST) / PARAM =REF;

                      MODEL P_YEAR*DEATH(0)= HFDM / RISKLIMITS ;

                      BASELINE COVARIATES=REG_HFDM OUT=_NULL_;

                          RUN;

                  ODS GRAPHICS OFF;
```

Output

The results (Fig. 5.8) show that patients with heart failure and diabetes had the poorest survival probability (line 3 in brown) and those without heart failure and diabetes had the best survival probability (line 0 in blue).

Analysis of Maximum Likelihood Estimates

Parameter		DF	Parameter Estimate	Standard Error	Chi-Square	$P>$ChiSq	Hazard Ratio	95% Hazard Ratio Confidence Limits		Label
HFDM	1	1	0.60464	0.06663	82.3359	<.0001	1.831	1.606	2.086	HFDM 1
HFDM	2	1	0.93710	0.09402	99.3499	<.0001	2.553	2.123	3.069	HFDM 2
HFDM	3	1	1.43268	0.12681	127.6431	<.0001	4.190	3.268	5.372	HFDM 3

The hazards ratios (HRs) show a clear "dose-response" relationship between patients with different disease status (joint with or without diabetes in patients with or without heart failure) and the risk of all-cause mortality. It indicates that, compared with the reference group (i.e., those without heart failure and diabetes), patients

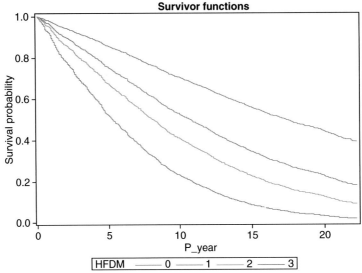

FIG. 5.8 Survival probability by heart failure (HF) and diabetes mellitus (DM) status.

with both heart failure and diabetes had 4.19 times higher risk of death (95%CI: 3.268–5.372, $P<.0001$). The HRs (95%CIs) of those with heart failure only for all-cause mortality was 2.553 (2.123–3.069), and the HRs (95%CI) of those with diabetes only for all-cause mortality was 1.831 (1.606–2.086).

REFERENCES

1. Rothman K, Greenland D, Lash TL. *Modern Epidemiology.* vol. 3. Philadelphia, PA: Wolters Kluwer: Lippincott Williams and Wilkins; 2008.
2. Szklo M, Nieto FJ. *Epidemiology Beyond the Basics.* Vol. 2. Sudbury, MA: Jones and Bartlett; 2007.
3. Tabachnick Bg FLS. *Using Multivariate Statistics.* Vol. 5. Boston, MA: Allyn & Bacon; 2007.
4. Trapp BDaRG. *Basic & Clinical Biostatistics.* New York, NY 10041: McGraw-Hill Companies, Inc.; 2004.
5. Motulsky H. *Intuitive Biostatistics: A Nonmathematical Guide to Statistical Thinking.* USA: Oxford University Press; 2013.
6. Gordis L. *Epidemiology.* 5th ed. Toronto, Canada: Elsevier Canada; 2014.
7. David G, Kleinbaum MK. *Survival Analysis a Self-learing Text.* New York, USA: Springer; 2012.
8. Kaplan EL, Meier P. Nonparametric estimation from incomplete observations. *J Am Stat Assoc.* 1958;53(282): 457–481.
9. Wikipedia KM. Kaplan–Meier estimator. https://en.wikipedia.org/wiki/Kaplan%E2%80%93Meier_estimator.
10. Schoenfeld D. Partial residuals for the proportional hazards regression model. *Biometrika.* 1982:239–241.

CHAPTER 6

Precision Medicine and Areas for Further Research

CHALLENGES AND OPPORTUNITIES IN HEART FAILURE RESEARCH

With the increasing trend in aging population and the complexity of heart failure, we are facing a significant challenge to prevent and control the risk of heart failure.[1,2] There is no doubt that the incidence of heart failure, the number of patients with heart failure, and the number of death due to heart failure will be very likely to increase continuously. Heart failure will remain as one of the leading cause of death for the Americans and populations worldwide in the coming decades.

More studies with hypothesis-driven study designs and application of advanced biostatistical analysis approaches are needed.

PRECISION MEDICINE AND PRECISION PUBLIC HEALTH

Precision Medicine

Precision medicine is a term used to describe individualized treatment that encompasses the use of new diagnostics and therapeutics, targeted to the needs of a patient based on his/her own genetic, biomarker, phenotypic, or psychosocial characteristics. The recent development of large-scale biologic databases has made it possible to promote new concept and practice in precision medicine, for example, the human genome sequence project and newly developed robust methods for characterizing patients (i.e., proteomics, metabolomics, genomics, diverse cellular assays, and even mobile health technology) and computational tools for analyzing large sets of data.[3,4]

Precision Public Health

As precision medicine is about providing the right treatment to the right patient at the right time, a similar term, the precision public health, has been proposed. At the population level, precision public health is about providing the right intervention to the right population at the right time. It aims to improve the ability to prevent disease, promote health, and reduce health disparities in populations.[5]

The complexity of heart failure demonstrates the need for multidisciplinary studies. The integrating of both precision medicine at an individual level and the precision public health at community and population levels will play a pivotal role in control and prevention of heart failure.

AREAS FOR FURTHER RESEARCH

Prevention for People at High Risk of Health Failure

Patients at American College of Cardiology (ACC)/American Heart Association (AHA) stage A are at high risk of heart failure. Few studies have been conducted to estimate the burden and prediction of heart failure.

Hospitalized Heart Failure

Hospitalized heart failure (HHF) is the leading cause of hospitalization in the United States. Although the per capita HHF rate may be beginning to decline in the United States, the early postdischarge mortality and readmission rates have remained largely unchanged and may even be worsening.[6,7] However, there is currently an unmet critical need in HHF to design and conduct rational, global, hospital-based registries to better understand this heterogeneous patient population, inform public policy decisions, and guide basic, translational, and clinical research.[8]

Multicomorbidity and Cardiorenal Failure

The severity of multiple comorbidities in patients with heart failure is well known, although the etiologic association is largely unknown. Given an increasing number of patients with chronic kidney disease, further studies with focusing on multicomorbidities in patients with heart failure are needed.[9–11]

Cardiometabolic Syndrome and Heart Failure

Given an increasing prevalence of obesity and prevalence of diabetes, the relationship between cardiometabolic syndrome and risk of heart failure needs to be further studied.[12–14]

Therapies and Polypharmacy in Patients With Heart Failure

Multicomorbidities and polypharmacy exist together, and their interaction on the outcomes of heart failure needs to be further studied.[15,16] HHF is an opportune time to review current management and implement evidence-based therapies for chronic heart failure in a controlled and monitored setting; indeed, in-hospital initiation of therapy is one of the best predictors of long-term use.[17–19]

Readmission in Patients With Heart Failure

A continuously high readmission rates in patients with heart failure causes a severe burden of the unitization of healthcare resources locally and nationally.[20] In the OPTIMIZE-HF (Organized Program to Initiate Lifesaving Treatment in Hospitalized Patients With Heart Failure) study with follow-up cohort representing about 10% of the overall registry, the readmission rate was approximately 30% within 60–90 days postdischarge and mortality ranged from 5.4% to 14.0% based on admission systolic blood pressure. Similarly, the ESC-HF (European Society of Cardiology–Heart Failure) Pilot Survey reported 1-year mortality and readmission rates of 17.4% and 31.9%, respectively, at representative centers from 12 European countries.[8,21] Limited data are available to identify the causes of readmission regarding its association with quality of care, current health policy, and health insurance system.[22,23]

Biomarkers and Prediction Models in Patients With Heart Failure

The interest in biomarker measures and studies can be back to the mid-1950s, and serum C-reactive protein was found to be related an increased risk of heart failure. Inflammation and risk of heart failure have been paid a considerable attention. However, several other biomarkers may add new evidence to diagnosis and prediction of the disease progress.[24–26] For example, the OPTIMIZE-HF registry found that eight factors, including age, weight, systolic blood pressure, sodium, serum creatinine, and comorbid disease states, could predict the combined endpoint of death or readmission with a C-index of 0.72 (C-index, sometimes called the "concordance" statistic, is a measure of goodness of fit for binary outcomes in a logistic regression model. Values over 0.7 indicate a good prediction model. A value of 1 means that the model perfectly predicts those group members who will experience a certain outcome and those who will not).[27] The combination of an elevated B-type NP (natriuretic peptide) and positive troponin (Tn) levels (i.e., defined as TnI ≥1.0 ng/mL or TnT ≥0.1 ng/mL) in the ADHERE (Acute Decompensated Heart Failure National Registry) designated a small subset of patients (i.e., ~5%) who were at a particularly high risk for short-term mortality.[28] The most widely accepted independent predictors of morbidity and mortality in HHF patients include age, cardiac and noncardiac comorbidities, systolic blood pressure, renal function (i.e., blood urea nitrogen and serum creatinine), serum sodium, hemoglobin, NP concentration, troponin, QRS duration, and evidence-based medication utilization.[8]

However, the most studies of biomarkers in heart failure patients focus on biologic biomarkers, these studies did not address or paid less attention to lifestyle factors, environmental factors, and few of them paid attention to socioeconomic and health policy relevant determinants of the development of heart failure. A comprehensive strategy of control and prevention of heart failure must focus both precision medicine and precision public health (including health policy).

Reverse Epidemiology of Heart Failure

Reverse epidemiology is one of the most important concepts and theories in chronic disease epidemiology.[29–31] Findings from several observational epidemiologic studies suggest that classical cardiovascular risk factors, such as body mass index (BMI), total cholesterol, and systolic blood pressure, are associated with improved, rather than impaired, survival in heart failure ("reverse epidemiology"), specifically in older adults with severe heart failure. For example, in a cohort study of patients with heart failure (n = 867; mean [SD] age, 70 [±13] years), risk of mortality counterintuitively increased on a cumulative scale with lower levels of BMI, total cholesterol, and systolic blood pressure, irrespective of the type and severity of heart failure.[32] A reverse association between all-cause mortality and patients with a decreased BMI was observed in our early studies as well.[33,34] The underlying mechanism by which factors that may contribute to the reverse association is largely unknown. Patients with heart failure have a high proportion of those with kidney dysfunction or with end stage renal disease (ESRD). Both the conditions share many clinical and pathophysiological aspects. They comprise patient groups suffering from a severe and similar burden of comorbidities, as anemia, malnutrition, diabetes, and other cardiovascular risk factors (or called cardiorenal syndrome) that may mutually contribute to disease progression and may partly explain the paradox of reverse epidemiology in patients with severe heart failure. Future studies need to identify whether risk factor control, as presently recommended, should be advocated in all patients with heart failure.[32]

Impact of Big Data on Heart Failure Study

The rapidly expanding field of big data analytics has started to play a pivotal role in the evolution of healthcare practices and research. Big data can help us compute missing probabilities and inform rational decisions across demographic groups that are underrepresented in past studies.[35] However, possible misleading due to the selection of an inappropriate method of analysis and/or the quality of big data may occur. Researchers should be aware of this and minimize the potential pitfalls.[36,37]

REFERENCES

1. Rich MW. Heart failure in older adults. *Med Clin North Am.* 2006;90(5):863–885.xi.
2. Stewart S, MacIntyre K, Capewell S, McMurray JJ. Heart failure and the aging population: an increasing burden in the 21st century? *Heart.* 2003;89(1):49–53.
3. Collins FS, Varmus H. A new initiative on precision medicine. *N Engl J Med.* 2015;372(9):793–795.
4. Jameson JL, Longo DL. Precision medicine–personalized, problematic, and promising. *N Engl J Med.* 2015;372(23):2229–2234.
5. Khoury MJ, Iademarco MF, Riley WT. Precision public health for the era of precision medicine. *Am J Prev Med.* 2016;50(3):398.
6. Blecker S, Paul M, Taksler G, Ogedegbe G, Katz S. Heart failure–associated hospitalizations in the United States. *J Am Coll Cardiol.* 2013;61(12):1259–1267.
7. Liu L. Changes in cardiovascular hospitalization and comorbidity of heart failure in the United States: findings from the National Hospital Discharge Surveys 1980–2006. *Int J Cardiol.* 2011;149(1):39–45.
8. Ambrosy AP, Fonarow GC, Butler J, et al. The global health and economic burden of hospitalizations for heart failure: lessons learned from hospitalized heart failure registries. *J Am Coll Cardiol.* 2014;63(12):1123–1133.
9. Gil P, Justo S, Caramelo C. Cardio-renal failure: an emerging clinical entity. *Nephrol Dial Transplant.* 2005;20(9):1780–1783.
10. McCullough PA, Hassan SA, Pallekonda V, et al. Bundle branch block patterns, age, renal dysfunction, and heart failure mortality. *Int J Cardiol.* 2005;102(2):303–308.
11. Coresh J, Selvin E, Stevens LA, et al. Prevalence of chronic kidney disease in the United States. *JAMA.* 2007;298(17):2038–2047.
12. Li C, Ford ES, McGuire LC, Mokdad AH. Association of metabolic syndrome and insulin resistance with congestive heart failure: findings from the Third National Health and Nutrition Examination Survey. *J Epidemiol Community Health.* 2007;61(1):67–73.
13. Owan TE, Redfield MM. Epidemiology of diastolic heart failure. *Prog Cardiovasc Dis.* 2005;47(5):320–332.
14. Vaur L, Gueret P, Lievre M, Chabaud S, Passa P, study DSG. Development of congestive heart failure in type 2 diabetic patients with microalbuminuria or proteinuria: observations from the DIABHYCAR (type 2 DIABetes, Hypertension, CArdiovascular Events and Ramipril) study. *Diabetes Care.* 2003;26(3):855–860.
15. Wong CY, Chaudhry SI, Desai MM, Krumholz HM. Trends in comorbidity, disability, and polypharmacy in heart failure. *Am J Med.* 2011;124(2):136–143.
16. Lien CT, Gillespie ND, Struthers AD, McMurdo ME. Heart failure in frail elderly patients: diagnostic difficulties, comorbidities, polypharmacy and treatment dilemmas. *Eur J Heart Fail.* 2002;4(1):91–98.
17. Gattis WA, O'Connor CM, Gallup DS, Hasselblad V, Gheorghiade M, Investigators I-H. Predischarge initiation of carvedilol in patients hospitalized for decompensated heart failure: results of the Initiation Management Predischarge: Process for Assessment of Carvedilol Therapy in Heart Failure (IMPACT-HF) trial. *J Am Coll Cardiol.* 2004;43(9):1534–1541.
18. Albert NM, Fonarow GC, Abraham WT, et al. Predictors of delivery of hospital-based heart failure patient education: a report from OPTIMIZE-HF. *J Card Fail.* 2007;13(3):189–198.
19. Butler J, Arbogast PG, Daugherty J, Jain MK, Ray WA, Griffin MR. Outpatient utilization of angiotensin-converting enzyme inhibitors among heart failure patients after hospital discharge. *J Am Coll Cardiol.* 2004;43(11):2036–2043.
20. Gwadry-Sridhar FH, Flintoft V, Lee DS, Lee H, Guyatt GH. A systematic review and meta-analysis of studies comparing readmission rates and mortality rates in patients with heart failure. *Arch Intern Med.* 2004;164(21):2315–2320.
21. Sliwa K, Hilfiker-Kleiner D, Mebazaa A, et al. EURObservational research programme: a worldwide registry on peripartum cardiomyopathy (PPCM) in conjunction with the heart failure association of the European Society of Cardiology Working Group on PPCM. *Eur J Heart Fail.* 2014;16(5):583–591.
22. Hunt SA, Abraham WT, Chin MH, et al. 2009 focused update incorporated into the ACC/AHA 2005 Guidelines for the diagnosis and management of heart failure in adults: a report of the American College of Cardiology Foundation/American Heart Association Task Force on practice Guidelines: developed in collaboration with the International Society for Heart and Lung Transplantation. *Circulation.* 2009;119(14):e391–e479.
23. Yancy CW, Abraham WT, Albert NM, et al. Quality of care of and outcomes for African Americans hospitalized with heart failure: findings from the OPTIMIZE-HF (organized program to initiate Lifesaving treatment in hospitalized patients with heart failure) registry. *J Am Coll Cardiol.* 2008;51(17):1675–1684.
24. Tousoulis D, Kampoli AM, Siasos G, et al. Circulating biomarkers for the diagnosis and prognosis of heart failure. *Curr Med Chem.* 2009;16(29):3828–3840.
25. Tribouilloy C, Rusinaru D, Leborgne L, Peltier M, Massy Z, Slama M. Prognostic impact of angiotensin-converting enzyme inhibitor therapy in diastolic heart failure. *Am J Cardiol.* 2008;101(5):639–644.

26. Braunwald E. Biomarkers in heart failure. *N Engl J Med.* 2008;358(20):2148–2159.

27. O'connor CM, Abraham WT, Albert NM, et al. Predictors of mortality after discharge in patients hospitalized with heart failure: an analysis from the organized program to initiate lifesaving treatment in hospitalized patients with heart failure (OPTIMIZE-HF). *Am Heart J.* 2008;156(4):662–673.

28. Giamouzis G, Kalogeropoulos A, Georgiopoulou V, et al. Hospitalization epidemic in patients with heart failure: risk factors, risk prediction, knowledge gaps, and future directions. *J Card Fail.* 2011;17(1):54–75.

29. Kalantar-Zadeh K, Anker SD, Horwich TB, Fonarow GC. Nutritional and anti-inflammatory interventions in chronic heart failure. *Am J Cardiol.* 2008;101(11A): 89E–103E.

30. Oreopoulos A, Padwal R, Kalantar-Zadeh K, Fonarow GC, Norris CM, McAlister FA. Body mass index and mortality in heart failure: a meta-analysis. *Am Heart J.* 2008;156(1):13–22.

31. Horwich TB, Fonarow GC. Reverse epidemiology beyond dialysis patients: chronic heart failure, geriatrics, rheumatoid arthritis, COPD, and AIDS. *Seminars Dialysis.* 2007;20(6):549–553.

32. Guder G, Frantz S, Bauersachs J, et al. Reverse epidemiology in systolic and nonsystolic heart failure: cumulative prognostic benefit of classical cardiovascular risk factors. *Circ Heart Fail.* 2009;2(6):563–571.

33. Liu L, Bopp MM, Roberson PK, Sullivan DH. Undernutrition and risk of mortality in elderly patients within 1 year of hospital discharge. *J Gerontol A Biol Sci Med Sci.* 2002;57(11):M741–M746.

34. Sullivan DH, Liu L, Roberson PK, Bopp MM, Rees JC. Body weight change and mortality in a cohort of elderly patients recently discharged from the hospital. *J Am Geriatr Soc.* 2004;52(10):1696–1701.

35. Belle A, Thiagarajan R, Soroushmehr S, Navidi F, Beard DA, Najarian K. Big data analytics in healthcare. *BioMed Res Int.* 2015;2015.

36. Deo RC, Nallamothu BK. Learning about machine learning: the promise and pitfalls of big data and the electronic health record. *Circ Cardiovasc Qual Outcomes.* 2016;9(6):618–620.

37. Ahmad T, Testani JM, Desai NR. Can big data simplify the complexity of modern medicine?: prediction of right ventricular failure after left ventricular assist device support as a test case. *JACC Heart Fail.* 2016;4(9):722–725.

Index

'Note: Page numbers followed by "f" indicate figures and "t" indicate tables.'